CW01618730

Losing My Voice!

Living with Motor Neurone Disease

Barbara Frances Williams

NZRGON, MHSc. (Hons)

First published August 2007
Publishers: publishing@kevinz. Auckland

ISBN 978-0-473-12488-5

Book and cover designed by Kevin Williams
Photographs: from family snapshots

For all those recently diagnosed with MND/ALS
and those yet to be diagnosed, wishing that
my story may provide inspiration and hope.

Motor Neurone Disease (MND)

Motor neurone disease (MND) also known as amyotrophic lateral sclerosis (ALS) is a progressive neurological condition where motor neurones are destroyed. Motor neurones are the cells that control voluntary muscle activity such as speaking, walking, hand movement, talking, breathing, and swallowing. Symptoms of MND may begin in one area of the body but will progress to other areas. As the disease progresses help is needed to carry out activities of daily living such as self care and feeding. MND is usually fatal within 2-5 years and 50% will die within 14 months of diagnosis. Only one in five will survive for five years. Death is usually due to respiratory (breathing) failure.

About 90% of cases of MND/ALS are "sporadic," meaning that the person has no family history of it.

Emotional lability / pseudobulbar effect: about one third of MND sufferers experience emotional lability in the form of crying and pathological laughter.

Acknowledgements

To Margie and the Multidisciplinary MND team at Prince of Wales and Calvary Hospitals, Sydney, and Caroline at the NSW MND Assn, thanks for your expert care. Special thanks to Margie for going the 'extra mile' and to Patsy who came to my 'rescue' when I was locked out!

To the unknown members of the public whose assistance and acts of kindness are mentioned in this book, thanks!

To Michael and the team at Soul Pharmacy Railway Parade, the team at the Kogarah Commonwealth Bank and Karmyn at the gym, thanks for your patience while I wrote down what I wanted to say.

To the following special people who each in their own way have helped me cope, have provided encouragement, support, friendship and most of all have kept on talking to me regardless, THANKS!

Mary and Sheila who have encouraged me to keep writing. Special thanks to Mary for proof reading, and to Marcia and Barbara for editing.

Carol, Bronwyn, Pauline, Chris, Linda, Robyn, Robyn and Robyn (yes, three Robyns), John, Harvey and all of my friends and former colleagues.

The doctors, research coordinators and administrative staff at the many hospitals in Australia and New Zealand that I visited in the course of my work.

The team at PCRG Ross, Jennifer, Jo, Trish and Tyron.

And to Barbara, my oldest friend, and to my family, Kevin, Dylan, Emma, Aaliyah, Mum, Jenni and Francis, Gavin and Debra, special thanks for your love and support - what would I have done without you?

Contents

Preface

I am conscious that in telling my story I make only passing reference to individual members of my family. This is intentional. This is not a story about my family. Over the years we have come to value our privacy. This story is but one of the many chapters in my life. It is a story about how I am affected by, and cope with, the devastating, incurable and rapidly fatal condition known as motor neurone disease (MND). I make passing reference to events that have shaped my character and perhaps will help the reader to understand the manner in which I cope with the illness.

Shortly after I was diagnosed with MND I began to think that maybe I should write down what was happening to me. I didn't have any particular end in sight. Maybe I would write a paper for publication in a nursing, medical or ethics journal. Maybe I would write a book. Or maybe I would just write something for my family to read so that they could understand what was happening to me.

I very quickly found and read medical papers on all aspects of MND, its diagnosis and treatment. Books and papers on euthanasia and associated ethical aspects were also easy to come by. Then as time went on I began to find newspaper articles and books written by or about people with MND recounting their experiences and thoughts as they cope with the impact of the disease. Many of these are referred to in parts of this book.

Because I wrote about most of the events described in this book as they were happening or shortly afterwards, I have mainly written in the present tense. I have tried to be as accurate as possible in recounting conversations that took place. Most of the medical professionals whose consultations are described in this book remain nameless to preserve their privacy and professional reputation. I have not set out to be judgmental. I have described things as they happened to me and how I was affected and where appropriate I mention what I think should have happened. I must point out that all the medical professionals that I consulted were aware of my health professional background at the time the consultations took place.

I would also like to point out that I am not wallowing in self pity. People who have known me over this time know that I just got on with my busy life with a reasonably positive outlook.

There are several things that I hope this book will achieve. Firstly that people may gain an increased awareness of MND, the disease itself and some of the ethical issues associated with the disease.

Secondly that by revealing some of the difficulties I have encountered both physically and emotionally, and the distressing experiences I have had with some of my medical consultations, that I may provide some insight and be a catalyst for change so that people might appreciate how seemingly little things may have enormously negative impacts on patients when they are vulnerable.

Once diagnosed with MND, there is currently no hope of a cure. The best one can hope for is to slow the progression of the disease. People may react in several ways to the diagnosis of motor neurone disease. They can devote themselves to fighting the disease, they can try to live as fully as they can or they can give up. I am trying to live as fully as I can while I am able to. This is my story.

1
Early Life

The circumstances of my birth were eloquently described by my father in his book *The Rise and Fall of a Young Turk*:

> We were fortunate that Barbara was born prematurely and although badly jaundiced survived through, we fondly believe, a certain innate toughness which has stood this small girl in good stead on various subsequent occasions. She was born at the old Narrow Neck camp hospital and during her premature birth the table on which she was being delivered began to collapse. It was held up by a nursing sister with a back ailment who suffered a long and painful ordeal until the baby was safely delivered. She would perhaps feel happy to know that from the age of four Barbara had no other thought than to be a nurse - and so it was.[1]

And so it was. At the age of seventeen I began my nursing training at Wellington Hospital.

My early life and character was undoubtedly influenced by my father's political career and the resulting moves from our original family home in Devonport to Kohimarama and then to Wellington. I found the moves to new schools unsettling and did not make new friends quickly.

As a child, each winter, I suffered bouts of respiratory infections labeled 'bronchitis' by the family doctor. In those days the 'times tables' were learned by rote with the whole class sitting on the mat and chanting "5 x 5 is 25, 5 x 6 is 30" etc. Several times I remember returning to school after a bout of bronchitis to find that I had missed learning a 'times table.' My spelling also suffered but not to the same extent as my arithmetic. I don't ever remember being encouraged to catch up on the school work that I had missed.

Being left handed my handwriting was untidy. When I started school as a five year old my teacher would take the chalk from my left hand and place it in my right hand. As soon as her back was turned I swapped the chalk back to my left hand and I have remained firmly left handed. In those days teachers expected pupils to have neat handwriting that conformed to the style of the day; my left handed style did not. I remember when I was in Standard three my zealous teacher, who thought that my style of handwriting would hinder me in adult life, often kept me in after school to practise my handwriting.

I moved from primary school to secondary school thinking that I was not very bright. This feeling was reinforced by being placed in the bottom of the two third form classes at Wellington's Marsden School. Throughout my secondary school years, however, I did reasonably well academically but I never really enjoyed school. I worked hard to pass the exams on the first attempt and to leave school as soon as I could. I had no desire to go on to university, wanting only to leave school and have a 'paying job.'

Nursing fitted the bill. As my father noted, I had long thought of nursing as a career, however an important factor in my choice was that I would be gaining a qualification whilst working and receiving a regular pay packet. In May 1969 I entered the Wellington Hospital School of Nursing as a student nurse. Initially we worked a six day week and were moved to a different ward every six weeks. Again I found this constant change unsettling and I did not really enjoy my time as a student nurse. Determined to complete my training in the minimum period of three years I worked hard and became a registered nurse in June 1972.

I have always felt a sense of urgency to do things and a week after my final nursing exams I was married. My sister had introduced me to Kevin, who was a fellow student at the Wellington Polytechnic. In those days it was rather scandalous for a guy and girl to 'live together' and even more so for the daughter of a prominent politician, so we married and moved to Auckland.

I started work in ward 27, a men's medical ward at Auckland Hospital. The Coronary Care Unit was located at the end of that ward and it was not long before I was required to relieve the sole staff nurse in the Unit at meal times. Initially I was petrified of being left alone there with five sick and potentially unstable coronary patients. However, I soon found myself rostered to work full duties in the Coronary Care Unit and began to enjoy the work. In 1974 I completed a six month in-service certificate in coronary care nursing and surprised myself by coming top of the class of five.

In June 1975 at the age of twenty three I was appointed to the position of Ward Sister (later re-named Charge Nurse) of the Coronary Care Unit at Green Lane Hospital. I thoroughly enjoyed my five and a half years as Charge Nurse. The stability gave me confidence and security.

Kevin was born with a congenital degenerative bone condition and we were concerned that it could be passed on to any children that we might have, so in 1980 we adopted a baby boy whom we named Dylan and two years later we adopted Emma.

I never felt comfortable about not working and having an income of my own and for most of the time while the children were small I worked part time, firstly in the Coronary Care Unit at Green Lane Hospital and then in the Coronary Care Unit at North Shore Hospital.

In November 1987 Dr Robin Norris, who was the physician in charge of the Coronary Care Unit at Green Lane Hospital and my former boss, asked me if I would like to come and help him with his research for a few weeks. Shortly after this Emma turned five and started school and I continued 'helping' with the research on a part time basis. In time part time stretched to become full time, Robin Norris moved to England and Harvey White became the Director of the Cardiovascular Research Unit at Green Lane

Hospital. Fifteen and a half years later the staff of the research unit had grown to more than twenty and as manager of the acute trials section of the unit I was still 'helping' with the research.

1 Muldoon, R.D. (1974) *The Rise and Fall of a Young Turk*. (p. 22). A.H. & A.W. Reed: Wellington. www.reed.co.nz - Reproduced with permission given by Reed Publishing (NZ) Ltd.

2

Moving to Sydney and early symptoms

I moved to Sydney in June 2003 to take up a job as a Clinical Research Associate (CRA) with the Australian affiliate of a large American pharmaceutical company. The decision to leave my job in Auckland where for 15 or so years I had worked as a Clinical Trials Coordinator was not made without a lot of thought. Over the years I had taken on increasing responsibility and by and large been very happy. For several years, though, I had been thinking about working as a CRA. The timing, however, was never right. Something always seemed to take priority: I was working on an exciting trial, I had started my part time study towards a Master's degree, or my daughter Emma was having a baby. After completing my Master of Health Science Degree (awarded with first class honours) in 2001, and subsequently having my thesis research published in the prestigious medical journal *Lancet*, I now feel that I have reached a glass ceiling in my job at Green Lane Hospital and decide that I am finally ready for a new challenge.

It's not easy for a middle aged woman to apply for and be appointed to a CRA position. I apply for a dozen or so jobs, firstly for jobs in Auckland and then in Sydney. I am always interviewed but the feedback in rejection letters hints that I am either too experienced or, as I have always worked in Cardiology, that I am too specialised. Later I learn that some prospective employers thought that I was just 'testing the waters' and was not serious about wanting a new job. Others who had collaborative research links with our research unit did not want to 'poach' me. So I am elated to finally be offered a one year contract as a Sydney based CRA, with the added bonus of a salary substantially higher than my hospital nurse's salary.

I resign, giving one month's notice, and start to make plans to move to Sydney. My husband Kevin and son Dylan will remain in the family home in Auckland, Emma is living happily with her partner and daughter in West Auckland and I will come home when I can for weekends and holidays. For some time I have been talking to my extended family about wanting to get a job in Sydney so when I actually get the job it does not come as a complete surprise.

On June 16 2003 with one suitcase of belongings, I board a plane to Sydney. On arrival at Sydney airport the immigration official is more interested in how I have completed my SARS (sudden acute respiratory syndrome) questionnaire than in the category 'A' (migrating to Australia) immigration status entered on my arrival card. I check into a hotel a few minutes away from my new job and two days later I start work. Within 10 days I have bought a car and leased and furnished an apartment in Kogarah, South Sydney. Knowing that a CRA is required to travel frequently by air to research sites, I choose to live close to Sydney airport. Six weeks later three boxes of household goods and clothes arrive by sea from Auckland and I begin to feel at home.

My apartment in Kogarah is ideal. It is brand new. From my sixth floor balcony I have a wonderful view of Sydney's Botany Bay, the airport, container terminal and on the far side of the bay, the oil refinery and the national park. There is underground security parking. It is a three minute walk to the shopping centre and the railway station and for $3.60 (return) I can reach downtown Sydney by train in 20 minutes. Work is one hour away by car. Driving one hour each way to and from work every day, getting to grips with a new job and frequently travelling inter-state, my life is busy and I don't really have time to worry about any possible health problems.

During this time I have a dry cough and at times a husky voice which becomes worse as the day progresses. I put this down to the stress associated with my move and the new job and I assume that in time it will settle down. In January 2004 my daughter Emma, her partner Aaron and their daughter Aaliyah spend a week with me in Sydney. This is when I first notice difficulty in swallowing and occasional slurred speech. On one occasion Emma, Aaron, Aaliyah and I are eating dinner on the balcony of my apartment enjoying a balmy Sydney evening and the panoramic view of Botany Bay. Suddenly I choke on a mouthful of wine and a spray of wine shoots out of my mouth and nose onto the tiles. Everyone laughs and they probably think that I have had too much to drink.

As the year progresses there are subtle changes. Food and fluids start to get stuck in my throat and I have increasing difficulties with my speech with occasional slurring of words and a husky nasal sounding voice. I have increasing cramps in my legs, toes and chest muscles. Despite getting plenty of sleep I yawn at inappropriate times during the day. And the cough continues. These changes are subtle and really I am unaware of the increasing nature of the symptoms or the significance of them.

Sometime in May a small advertisement in the *Sydney Morning Herald* catches my eye. "Experienced CRA required to join a dynamic CRO" the advertisement reads. "Must have significant experience as a site monitor with experience in cardiology trials." Although my one year contract has been extended to December 2004 my heart is still in cardiology and I decide to make inquiries about the advertised position. In mid June 2004 I am offered and accept the position of Senior CRA with a boutique contract research organization specializing in 'first in man' interventional cardiology trials. Initially I am hesitant about this home-based position, my major fear being the lack of technical IT support. My fears, however, are unfounded and in my new job, as with the previous one, I hit the ground running, and am 'full on' busy from day one.

3
Diagnosis and initial care

In August 2004 I finally decide to see a doctor about my ongoing cough and husky voice. The general practitioner thinks that I might have a growth on my vocal cords and refers me to an Ear Nose and Throat (ENT) surgeon.

I see the ENT surgeon in his private rooms on August 17th. "I have a dry cough and a husky voice" I tell him. "I don't hear a cough" he remarks and quickly seems to dismiss this symptom. He doesn't ask me if I have any other symptoms, instead he says "Let's have a look at your vocal cords" and takes me into another room. After anaesthetising my throat with cocaine spray he threads a black tube through my nose and into my throat. He asks me to count from eighty to ninety and watches my vocal cords with the fiber optic scope. "I can see what the problem is" he says. "Your vocal cords are not closing properly when you speak. It's a common problem and it's easily fixed. I'd like you to see the speech therapist." The consultation had lasted about 15 minutes. *At least it's something that can be fixed.* I think as I make my way home.

I arrive on time for my first visit to the speech clinic at the public hospital and I wait for one and a half hours. The same ENT surgeon, this time in the company of his registrar and several medical students and the speech therapist, examines my vocal cords again with another fiber optic scope. They all watch my vocal cords on the video screen as I talk, repeating words they tell me. Then the surgeon asks me to explain my symptoms to the students. "For some time –" I start to say. The surgeon interrupts "When patients say 'for some time' they mean three or four months" "NO! three years" I correct him. I mention my cough and he says "But you came to see me about your voice." "Both the cough and the voice" I say as I thrust a list of my symptoms at him. He takes it, scans the bullet points and hands the list to his registrar saying sarcastically "Make 10 copies and put them in her notes!"

The following week I attend my first speech therapy session. The speech therapist asks me to explain my symptoms. By this stage I am feeling quite vulnerable and I am unable to speak without crying. I am given some voice exercises to do and I am asked to return a week or so later. At the next appointment the speech therapist asks me to perform various facial movements and gets me to move my tongue around and pull my tongue in and out rapidly. "Have you had any neurological problems?" she asks. "Not that I know of" I reply. "I think you need to see a neurologist" she adds.

A few weeks later, on October 19th I see a Sydney neurologist in his private rooms. After a quick physical examination the doctor says "You have a bulbar palsy and we need to see what is causing it. I would like you to have some blood tests. We need to see what's pressing on what - you need to have a MRI scan." There is no discussion of possible diagnoses and naturally with my limited neurological experience my first and lingering thought is that I have a brain tumour!

In between the doctors' appointments and the tests I continue working, travelling to hospitals in Melbourne, Auckland, Christchurch and Dunedin and returning in time for the next test or doctor's appointment. A few friends and colleagues have noticed the change in my speech and ask what is wrong. Mostly I say nothing and they go away thinking that perhaps I have had a stroke or something similar. A couple of friends are more persistent and manage to wheedle some details out of me. "You haven't got a brain tumor." "You are too well to have a brain tumour," they say when I voice my fears.

I have the blood tests and a few days later have the MRI scan. The MRI involves lying still while my head is inside the scanner.

For about 15 minutes the scanner whizzes and clicks and I have to keep still! This is hard to do. The more I try to keep still the more I want to wriggle and scratch imaginary itches. Also while I am lying flat saliva pools at the back of my throat and, unable to cough, I feel like I am choking. Between each recording I desperately try and swallow before the next request to take a breath and hold it. Finally the test is over and I wait a few more days for the results. On November 4th I return to the neurologist's rooms for the results.

Arriving at the consulting rooms five minutes before the appointment time I wait for forty five minutes. Firstly the consultation before mine runs over time. Then a lady and her husband walk in, without an appointment, with an x-ray that they want the neurologist to look at. The neurologist leaves his rooms with the x-ray to consult a radiographer and when he returns he discusses the x-ray findings with the lady and her husband. So by the time it is my turn, I enter the consulting room and sit down feeling neglected and vulnerable.

"The blood tests are OK and you don't have syphilis - we have to test for that" the neurologist says. "These are your MRI films" he says holding them up to the light box. "There is no sign of a brain tumour." *Oh* I think *maybe there's nothing wrong.*

"In view of the symptoms that you have, the physical findings of bulbar palsy," he continues "I think that you have Motor Neurone Disease." *Phew!* I think, *there is something wrong and I haven't been just imagining it. I'm not going mad.*

The relief is short lived. "Motor Neurone Disease" he continues "is a very serious disease. Half of the people with Motor Neurone Disease die within five years of diagnosis. But it is important to realise that the other half live longer than five years. The problems that you are having with swallowing and speaking will get worse and in time your respiratory muscles and arms and legs will be involved. I am going to start you on Riluzole. This is a drug that has been found to prolong the time to ventilation by about nine months. The good news is that you will retain control of your bladder and bowels."

Stunned, I sit there quietly sobbing while the neurologist phones to get the special authority approval number for the Riluzole. Riluzole is available in Australia under the Pharmaceutical Benefits Scheme (PBS). The full cost of the drug is AU$682.17 per month and under the PBS the patient only pays AU$28.60 a month. "Is this drug funded by Pharmac in New Zealand?" I ask. "No it isn't" he replies. "In New Zealand you will need to pay the full cost which will be almost NZ$10,000 per year."

"You have been crying a lot haven't you?" he comments. "The tendency to laugh or cry easily is part of this illness. If this doesn't settle down there is medication that can help. Do you have any questions?" Bewildered, I can't think. "Can I still drive my car?" I ask. "Yes" he replies. "I'd like to see you again in a month." And that was the end of the consultation. Barely 15 minutes to deliver a life shattering diagnosis. I had spent longer sitting in the waiting room than I did in his office.

Later from my reading of medical papers focusing on the management of MND I learn how much emphasis should be placed on giving the diagnosis. MND is a major and devastating life event and the diagnosis should be given with care and compassion. Over and over I read how patients complain of the hurried and insensitive manner in which they were told of their diagnosis.

It is stressed that the diagnosis of MND should be given caringly. Some indication of the possible diagnoses should be given. As considerable time may pass from the onset of symptoms until a person seeks a medical opinion and a diagnosis is made, it is suggested that patients are 'fast tracked' through the system to diagnosis. In my case despite initially seeing 'private' specialists it is 11 weeks from the time I am first seen by the ENT surgeon until I am given the diagnosis of MND.

For some of that time I have been away from Sydney working, however, if the ENT surgeon had taken a more detailed history of my symptoms and not jokingly brushed off my hand written list of symptoms and onset dates the alarm bells may have rung and my diagnosis been fast tracked. New Zealand neurologist Andrew

Chancellor, in an editorial in the *British Medical Journal* writes that patients often present with incompletely developed disease, and may be referred to variety of specialists. Changes in speech may lead to an ear, nose and throat referral.[1]

A State of the Art Lecture: *Workup of the Neurological Patient* by Gayle E Woodson MD mentions that speech changes in adults usually have a neurological cause. Patients with laryngeal dysfunction are difficult to diagnose because they often present to an ENT specialist rather than to a neurologist.[2]

Clearly then, my presentation and symptoms are fairly typical. I am surprised that an ENT specialist whom the GP that referred me said was 'the best in Sydney' did not consider the possibility of a neurological condition being the source of my speech and coughing problems. I wonder if I have a case for medical negligence but I don't have the will to pursue it. At the end of the day, nothing is going to make this dreadful disease go away.

With tears still in my eyes I pay for the consultation and walk the 20 minutes from Darlinghurst down Oxford Street to the Museum station to catch the train home. I am bewildered. Despite my long career as a nurse and research coordinator I know next to nothing about MND. I certainly have no idea of the horrors of the disease that I am about to discover.

Arriving home I log onto the internet and search for MND. I am stunned! *This disease is so awful you wouldn't wish it on your worst enemy!! What on earth am I going to do? How do I tell my family? I don't feel as though I have a terminal illness. They have made a mistake.* Thoughts race through my mind.

I can't stop crying. In the course of my internet searches I learn about the pseudo bulbar effect which is a condition characterised by frequent episodes of inappropriate laughing or crying that are out of proportion to the situation at hand and are common in MND with bulbar onset. Outbursts of crying or laughing can occur spontaneously or in response to stimuli such as questions or events.

A few days later I have another appointment with the speech therapist. “I’m not surprised” she says when I tell her what the diagnosis is. Although she had never given me any indication of what she thought might be wrong with me, the speech therapist has really been the most helpful health professional that I have seen so far. She gives me contact details for the New South Wales Motor Neurone Disease Association (NSW MND Assn.) and strongly advises me to make contact with them. *Why didn’t the neurologist tell me this?* I wonder.

As luck would have it the NSW Motor Neurone Disease Association is located on the site of Concord Hospital. One of my research sites is at Concord and I am due to go there only a couple of days later.

I walk into the Motor Neurone Disease Association office. “Can I help you?” a lady asks. Although I have walked into the office dressed professionally and full of confidence I immediately burst out in tears, great sobs, and I am quite incapable of speaking. She kindly ushers me over to another lady in the corner who offers me some tissues. There is no privacy in the open plan area. Slowly, between the sobs, I manage to say “I.........have........ Motor...Neurone.........” I manage to utter enough words so that by the end of 15 minutes or so I have given her my contact details and have asked for and been given some MND Association brochures to give to my family.

Things happen very quickly after that. I am visited at home by the MND Association Family Support Regional Advisor and I am put in contact with Margie, the Nurse Co-coordinator of the Multidisciplinary MND service. Margie visits me at home and arranges for me to attend the next Multidisciplinary MND clinic at Prince of Wales Hospital. This clinic is part of the public hospital system and provides a comprehensive service.

The following week I am due to be in Auckland for work so through my Auckland GP I arrange an appointment with an Auckland neurologist for a second opinion. In contrast with the brief neurological consultations that I had in Sydney the Auckland consultation is very thorough and lasts over one hour. The neurologist confirms the diagnosis of MND and also confirms that in New Zealand Riluzole is not currently and not likely to be funded by Pharmac. It is not even registered for use in New Zealand.

I spend the weekend at home in Auckland with my family. I know that I must tell them. But how do you tell your family that you have a terminal illness for which there is no cure? In the end it isn't as hard as I had feared. Kevin and I go to the local Japanese restaurant for dinner on the Friday night. "I have found out why I am coughing" I say cautiously. "I've got Motor Neurone Disease." "Ooooh …….. I know something about that" Kevin says quietly. "I saw a television programme last year about Dudley Moore when he had Motor Neurone Disease." Somehow we get through dinner and go home. Somehow over the weekend I manage to tell my mother and my friend Barbara from Christchurch who is also in Auckland for the weekend.

Back in Sydney on December 7th I attend the MND clinic at the Prince of Wales Hospital where a third neurological examination again confirms a diagnosis of MND. I am still unable to speak about my symptoms without crying. The emotional lability is a common feature of the progressive bulbar palsy form of MND. The treatment of choice for this is Amitriptyline. This is a tricyclic antidepressant. Amitriptyline has sedative effects and when taken at night aids sleep. It also helps to dry up saliva which can be a problem when swallowing is impaired. For me Amitriptyline has an immediate effect. I sleep better, and find that there is an improvement in my speaking and swallowing. But the crying doesn't stop.

At the clinic I also see the dietician, physiotherapist, occupational therapist and a social worker. At this stage I am active, fully mobile and totally independent and don't think that I need their services yet, however I am given sample packets of Sustagen, nutritional energy milk drink and recipes for soft easy-to-swallow food.

While I'm at the clinic I sign up for the Australian MND Registry. In formal terms I give informed consent for the medical details and progress of my disease to be recorded on a national data base. Participation in the registry is voluntary. The major focus of my Master's degree was on informed consent for participation in clinical trials. In my research work in Auckland I had a leading role in collecting and recording audit data on the treatment of heart disease so I wholeheartedly support this registry. Sometime later there is a short piece on the ABC news suggesting that MND should become a notifiable disease to enable compulsory collection of data. The news item features a former theatre nurse with MND who is filmed in a motorised wheel chair. There is still so much to learn about the causes, progress, treatment and possible cure of MND and compulsory collection of data will provide much needed information.

Throughout this time my working life carries on as usual. I continue to deal efficiently with work related issues without any problems or bouts of tears. However despite taking the Amitriptyline I am still prone to cry when talking about my symptoms or diagnosis.

Quite soon after my initial diagnosis I tell my boss by email, emphasising that I intend to continue working for as long as I can.

> Obviously I am devastated with the long term implications of this and I find it hard to talk about it without getting upset. I am very happy with my job and if I was asked to create the perfect CRA position for me - this would pretty much be it.

Fortunately his response is very supportive. I carry on with my busy schedule travelling to hospitals in Australia and New Zealand sometimes on a weekly basis, hoping that people will not notice my speech difficulty or ask too many questions.

I arrange my trips away from Sydney around my medical appointments.

Early in December my swallowing is formally assessed by a modified barium swallow. This is a test where you swallow food and fluids of varying consistencies that have been mixed with Barium. As the food or fluid is swallowed its progress down the gullet is captured by angiographic x-ray. The barium shows up on the moving x-ray picture. As I swallow the various substances I can clearly see the progress down the gullet on the TV screen. The substances take two or three swallows to completely leave the mouth and travel down the gullet. My swallowing is assessed as being 9/10 with 10 being normal.

Christmas is spent with my family in Auckland. I prepare Christmas dinner for my extended family at my mother's house wondering if this is the last Christmas that we will all be together. On New Year's Eve my granddaughter Aaliyah and her four year old cousin Raimana spend the night at my house. "Why do you talk funny?" asks Raimana. "There is something wrong with my voice" I reply.

I spend the first two weeks of the New Year with my mother on a South American Cruise. I happily realise that despite my illness I am much fitter than the majority of my fellow passengers who are mostly elderly North Americans. Many of the North American passengers have winter colds and as the cruise goes further south the bitterly cold weather forces us to stay inside and it becomes impossible to keep away from all the coughs and sneezes. Eventually I start to cough and sneeze too and my voice suffers and I find it hard to speak.

Arriving back in Sydney on 20 January 2005, I am straight back into my busy work routine and for each of the next four weeks I spend several days away from Sydney. Again I arrange my trips around my medical appointments.

On January 27th I have an Electromylogram (EMG) test. In this test electrodes are used to measure abnormal nerve and muscle activity. It's worse than going to the dentist! Firstly two electrodes are placed on an arm, one at each end of the forearm. Electrical currents, each one stronger than the previous one, are run from the upper electrode to the lower electrode making my arm jerk. This process is repeated on the other arm and then on each lower leg. The electric impulse feels like a very long, sharp, thin needle being forced rapidly down inside my arm or leg. When the tests are over the doctor says "Your left hand is weaker than your right one" "Yes, I know." I reply. "I have trouble opening things like bulldog clips with my left hand, yet I can do it easily with my right. And I am left handed! But I can still use chop sticks with my left hand." Immediately I think *what happens when I can't write?*

Next an acupuncture needle is inserted into various muscles, thumb, arm and leg and I am asked to tense the muscle as the readings are recorded on a computer. Then I have to lift my chin so that an acupuncture needle can be inserted through the skin under my jaw into my tongue! Then I am asked to touch the roof of my mouth with my tongue while the readings are recorded. Ouch! As I said, worse than going to the dentist!!

Later in the book *His Brother's Keeper* I read about Stephen Heywood's experience. His EMG lasted five hours. Needles were even inserted in his groin and painful electric shocks were delivered to his brain using an electrified skull cap.[3] By comparison I realise that I got off lightly with my test, but at the time I did not think so.

I drive home, have lunch and continue with my work until it's time to return to the hospital later in the afternoon for the appointment with the specialist respiratory physician.

In January I had caught a cold while I was away on a South American cruise with my mother and a few days earlier my cough had returned, and thus I have difficulty doing the breathing tests because every time I am instructed to blow hard, I cough.

Yet again I have floods of tears triggered by explaining my symptoms. The respiratory physician tells me that the cough is asthma. "However, your breathing muscles are working well and you won't stop breathing in the night!" He adds "If you want my two bob's worth, you should stop work and go back to Auckland to the care of your family." This only serves to intensify my distress as I reply "I was at home in Auckland for a week over Christmas and I was bored." After that I just can't control the tears. I have never cried uncontrollably like this in public before. I really wanted to say "If I go home I will be going home to die! And I'm not ready to do that." I need positive things to look forward to and I need to keep working for my own sanity.

A sleep test is arranged to assess my breathing while I sleep. This isn't much fun either. I am hooked up to so much gear that I can't get comfortable. There are electrocardiogram (ECG) electrodes (legs and shoulders and left chest). Because I sleep on that side the chest one keeps digging into me. Also, there are electroencephalogram (EEG) electrodes all over my head in my hair - luckily they don't cut any hair! As well there are two sets of nasal prongs, one metal and the other like plastic oxygen prongs but without oxygen, and a finger one too. "Is that thing staying on my finger all night?" I ask and the technician replies "Yes." "You'll be lucky" I reply. I have trouble going to sleep because the two staff keep talking for ages and I can't get comfortable. However, when I finally fall asleep, I sleep well.

"Sounds hideous," a medical colleague comments later, "but it sounds like normal sleeping conditions were ensured for your sleep test!" "I know that you're just having me on because you know more about these things than I do!" I reply. "A sleep test isn't a test to see how quickly you can fall asleep under extreme conditions. They should have been doing all they could to facilitate sleep." The following night I am relieved to be back at home in my own cosy bed.

In early March I attend an 'Ask the experts' day at Concord Hospital. This is put on by the NSW MND Association and includes an overview of MND, current therapies, theories and possibilities for treatments. There are updates on current research and information about the Australian MND DNA and tissue bank.

About a dozen people with various stages of MND have attended. Most are with a family member or care giver. I speak to the lady sitting next to me. "Why are you here?" she asks. Prompted by my hesitant reaction she asks "Do you have it?" "Yes" I reply. "It's my husband" she adds. "He's at home. What symptoms do you have?" Again I find it difficult to speak about what is happening to me. "My voice and swallowing," I murmur. Several people are in wheelchairs or have walking frames. Particularly distressing for me is one lady who is unable to move her arms or legs or to speak. *Is this is what is going to happen to me?* I wonder.

Current research in Australia seems to be at the basic science level. The presenter talks about there being an environmental and genetic interaction and affected people possibly have a gene mutation. In familial MND a mutant SOD 1 gene has been identified as being associated with the disease but it was emphasized that a mutant SOD 1 gene doesn't seem to be involved in sporadic MND which is what I have. Research is currently under way in Australia to collect blood for DNA analysis from people who are affected with MND and from controls who do not have the disease. During the day I give informed consent to be involved in the research and have a blood sample for DNA analysis taken.

Recently there has been some publicity about a New Zealand woman with bulbar palsy onset MND, who at the time of the 'ask the experts' meeting is in China awaiting implantation of stem cells into her brain. This procedure is highly controversial. I want to ask questions about stem cell therapy, but feel that I will not be able to ask the questions without crying. Fortunately while I am trying to pluck up the courage to ask, someone else asks the question. The response answers my questions. To date research with stem cells has been disappointing and has not been found to alter the course of the disease. The problems are where do you get the stem cells from? Where is the right place to insert the stem cells? Brain? Spinal cord? Blood? Once the stem cells are in place they keep dividing, and how do you stop them dividing? When cells keep dividing they can cause cancer. In China the stem cells are obtained from aborted fetuses. In most western countries this is a highly controversial source of stem cells.

At the moment there are no clinical trials with stem cells for the treatment of MND in Australia. However, in Sydney there is currently a clinical trial using stem cells for patients who have intractable cardiac ischemia. So maybe it is just a matter of time. However, for me I expect any advances will come too late.

Current research is focused on finding the cause of MND. Theories for the cause of sporadic MND involve exposure to various environmental contaminants and possibilities mentioned include heavy metals such as mercury, including dental fillings, toxins, organophosphates, a virus such as polio, or inflammatory causes. Intense physical training seems to be associated with MND as there is a high incidence of MND in professional footballers. In fact the young wife of a professional footballer who has MND was at this meeting. It was also suggested that stress might play a part. However, how and when do you measure stress and at what time point does the stress causing the disease occur? Not everyone who has had exposure to the environmental contaminants mentioned above gets MND thus it is postulated that those affected may have a mutant gene that makes them susceptible to developing the disease.

Also mentioned is the fact that the incidence of MND throughout the world is increasing although the reason for this is unknown. Possible reasons could be related to more precise methods of diagnosis and the ageing population.

A respiratory physician presents a case study describing the respiratory deterioration of a patient suffering from MND. He says that once overnight oxygen saturation level gets below 90% overnight ventilation using bi-level positive pressure (BiPAP) non-invasive ventilation is recommended. The rate of respiratory deterioration predicts survival and the use of overnight BiPAP has been shown to dramatically improve quality of life and survival. The case history focuses on the patient's respiratory deterioration, the side effects of prolonged ventilation, withdrawal of ventilation and death 14 hours later. I find this distressing. I think *I don't want this to happen. I don't want to die like this.*

Percutaneous Endoscopic Gastrostomy (PEG) is discussed. In many countries, including Australia, PEG is a standard procedure for maintaining adequate nutrition in people with impaired swallowing. Like BiPAP, PEG has been shown to dramatically improve quality of life and survival. The respiratory physician recommends three-monthly sleep tests to monitor respiratory status. He says that the timing of the introduction of BiPAP overnight ventilation and PEG is important and recommends that both are initiated during the same hospital admission. He mentions that survival after diagnosis is usually one-three years for bulbar palsy onset MND and that Riluzole prolongs survival by three-four months. This is a much shorter time than what I have been told at my initial diagnosis. Doing a quick mental calculation I think *I have probably had this for about 14 months already - I might only have a matter of months or a year or so left! I'm not ready for this and I certainly don't feel that ill.*

Later in March I go back to see the respiratory physician for a follow up to the sleep test. The breathing tests that I previously had difficulty doing are repeated. This time I am able to complete the tests without coughing. The results of the breathing tests are good. The doctor goes through the printed tracings of the sleep test. "This is during the rapid eye movement (REM) phase, when you are dreaming" he says. "See these smaller waves? These are periods of aponea. There aren't enough of these periods to be concerned about." Although not normal, the results are good enough so that I don't need to have overnight BiPAP ventilation. "I don't need to see you for six months" the doctor says. "In fact we could make it a year but I don't know how things will progress." I feel that is positive news, it gives me some sort of time frame and hope for the immediate future. "Are you going to carry on working and stay in Sydney?" he asks. "Yes" I reply. As I walk towards the door, he shakes my hand and says "Well things went a bit better this time; perhaps I was a bit confrontational last time?" "Thank you" I reply, unable to say more without crying.

1 Chancellor, Andrew M. (1996). *Diagnosing Motor Neurone Disease.* BMJ 1996; 312: 650-651.

2 Gayle E. Woodson. ALA: State of the Art Lecture: *Workup of the Neurolaryngology Patient.* www.alahns.org/trans/trans01/woodson.php Accessed 14 Oct 2006

3 Weiner J (2004). *His Brother's Keeper.* Harper Collins New York ISBN 0-06-001007-X

4

Telling friends and colleagues

Prior to my diagnosis various friends and colleagues who know me well had noticed a change in my voice. Several asked me what was wrong and quite honestly I could say "nothing" because I had not recently seen a doctor about my cough or voice changes. There were several reasons for this. Firstly it was difficult to take time off work to visit a doctor. I did not have medical insurance or a Medicare card in Australia. I had retained my New Zealand medical insurance policy and occasionally saw my Auckland GP. Because in New Zealand only people on low incomes are entitled to a Community Services card for discounted medical care, I mistakenly assumed that my income was too high for me to qualify for an Australian Medicare card. Somehow around about August 2004 I found out that everyone resident in Australia is entitled to have a Medicare card. So after living, working and paying tax in Australia for over one year I finally applied for and received a Medicare card. This opened the way for me to seek a diagnosis for my cough and voice changes.

Once I knew what was wrong with me I quickly resolved to put off telling people, other than immediate family, what was wrong. I had a hard enough time coming to terms with the implications of the diagnosis myself without wanting to be constantly subject to explanations and expressions of sympathy as I went about my work. Also I did not want colleagues to be constantly watching me for signs of deterioration, speculating on how much longer I could carry on, and waiting for me to die.

On one occasion while in Auckland I phoned a friend with the intention of telling her. However, she told me about another friend who had just been diagnosed with leukemia. I could tell from the tone of her voice that she was upset by the serious nature of our friend's illness and I didn't feel that I could burden her with further bad news.

Slurred or indistinct speech is not something you can hide. People who know me instantly notice the change in my voice and know that something is wrong. I am conscious that others who don't know me will judge me by my speech and possibly think that I have been drinking or that I am mentally handicapped. Thus as my voice deteriorates I feel that I can no longer hide things from the people I visit regularly in the course of my job.

Someone would ask "How are you?" Initially I replied "OK" but clearly something was wrong, so I tried to say "I have Motor Neurone Disease." However, each time I would start to cry and end up writing the words Motor Neurone Disease because I just couldn't say it. I hated breaking down in tears in the work situation so I developed a strategy of emailing one person at each research team who knew me well from my days as a study coordinator. I would explain the reason for my cough and voice change and ask them to quietly tell the rest of the team what was wrong.

Word got around, former colleagues and friends heard rumours and I couldn't hide it any longer. Unexpectedly I found the messages of understanding and support comforting.

Some messages of understanding and support

I will be honest I have heard a rumour that your health is still not good and I would love to be there for you if there is anything I can do.

I'm dismayed that I missed you on Thursday....... Your news came as a real bombshell. Like many others, I've been anxious about your health in recent months, but that's one formidable diagnosis. I guess it could never have come at a good time, but it's a shame that it should happen right when you're thriving in your job. It's good to know you have access to better treatment in Australia, though, and long may that continue.

> I am stunned and pissed off myself by your news and can only admire you for carrying on regardless. You are a brave lady.
>
> Lovely to hear from you, hang in there, feel free also to say you are pissed off. Would be nice to hear how you are getting on from time to time, with best regards and thoughts.
>
> SHIT!!!!! I am so sorry to hear that Barb.
>
> You are a brave lady and all of this is just bloody unfair.
>
> What dreadful news, a real bummer. Good on you for wanting to keep on in Oz. It's good that the drugs are covered there. NZ is so backward in these things. Hope work doesn't get too difficult for you though.
>
> Barb - I am really sorry to hear that - I can understand you wanting to keep working but shouldn't you be home with your friends and family for support? Who knows - maybe the Chinese treatment will be suitable for you - at least worth thinking about. Take care; it sounds as though you should slow down a bit.
>
> I am so sorry to hear such news and just wanted to let you know that you are in my thoughts and prayers.

By email I told an Adelaide-based colleague and friend who I had come to know over several years through our shared academic interest in informed consent. She writes:

> I am quite shocked by your news - when did you become aware that something was not right? It's hard to "discuss" this by email and I do hope you are in Adelaide soon so we can talk face to face. Are there any new therapies for motor neurone disease that you can try?

I reply:

> The best way for me to describe how I feel is "pissed off!" Over 2004 I started to get a husky voice and initially it was mis-diagnosed by an ENT surgeon who in retrospect did not "listen" to my history or examine me properly. It was the speech therapist who recognised that something else was wrong and had me referred to a Neurologist. I am on some very expensive

> medication that is available through the PBS, however in NZ Pharmac has refused to fund it. Anyway - I find it very difficult to talk about because really I am still physically very active - still go to the gym and don't feel or look sick. My boss is very supportive and I will keep working as long as I am able to. However, there will come a time that I can't carry on and will need to return to Auckland. At the moment my family realise that I need to just keep working. Cognitive function is not affected and I hope to be able to continue with some sort of work using my computer.

To which she replies:

> I think I would feel thoroughly pissed off too. I can understand that you want to keep working, and I guess it is important that you have access to this medication. You'll talk about it when you are ready to...if I can be of any help, you know where I am. Meanwhile...go girl!

One evening during a work trip to Auckland a friend who is recovering from breast cancer phones me. As she talks about her illness and mine I start to cry and just can't stop. After the call, in an effort to assure her that I was not an emotional cripple, I send her an email:

> Thanks for calling. I have been meaning to come and talk to you, knowing what you have been through but I just couldn't face the possibility of running into other people in the building. I am glad however, that I have had the opportunities that I have had in the last couple of years. I really am OK. I am certainly much better when I am working. Most of the sites that I visit now know what is wrong with my voice and they have been really supportive. The trouble is that emotional lability is part of the illness with the tendency to laugh or cry inappropriately.

Yes, the messages are comforting. Hopefully, people now realise that my slurred speech is not the result of an early morning drinking binge. Now I want to get on with living. I am not ready to die yet!

5
Grief - I'm not ready to die!

Joan Didion in her book *The Year of Magical Thinking* explores her own grief following the death of her husband and the serious illness of her only daughter. The waves of grief are not what she expects them to be. She writes of the choking, blinding paroxysms of grief that wipe out daily life.[1] There are times when I feel just like that. When I least expect it I am overcome by those same choking, blinding paroxysms of grief. I'm not scared of dying though. I expect that one night I'll just go to sleep and I won't wake up in the morning. I'm just not ready to die yet.

Throughout my adult life I have been very healthy, hardly taking any sick days off work. I am a non smoker. I don't have any known risk factors for heart disease and I have been taking prophylactic measures to prevent the onset of osteoporosis. Three of my grandparents lived until about the age of eighty, my paternal grandfather having died before I was born as a result of an illness contracted during World War I. Although my father died in his seventy first year my mother is fit and healthy at the age of seventy eight. Thus, I had every reason to expect to live until at least the age of eighty and I had planned and lived my adult life with that expectation.

The diagnosis of MND was therefore like a bolt from the blue. It was totally unexpected. Furthermore, in retrospect, I now realise that the manner in which I was informed of the diagnosis was inappropriate and insensitive and I feel that this has contributed to my ongoing grief.

I have worked in the health system all my adult life. I have daily communication as a health professional with medical colleagues.

I am able to read and objectively assess scientific papers on MND and its treatment and even to discuss the disease and its treatment in 'global terms' however, I continue to be unable to describe or discuss my own symptoms with the doctors treating me without crying.

Jonathan Warner captures my feelings exactly in the book *His Brother's Keeper* when he writes that there is a huge difference between asking questions as a professional and having a personal need for information. You are no longer the professional, in my case a nurse and clinical research associate, you are just a human being with a desperate need.[2]

I don't seem to be able to get past the denial stage. I know that I have MND. From my reading I am well aware of the clinical implications, the relentless progression of the disease and progress to eventual death. However, I feel fit, I'm active, go to the gym regularly and I certainly don't feel that I am dying! I don't accept that I'm dying! Sure, I have some difficulty swallowing and speaking and various painful muscle cramps. But they are all things that I can live with.

Strangely, in the six months since my diagnosis I have not been offered any counselling. I think that the Motor Neurone Disease Association family support regional advisor mentioned something about the possibility of counselling when she visited me but no one has been forthcoming with any offers of counselling. I don't know whether or not counselling would help. I am certainly not ready to accept the possibility of imminent death and I get upset thinking about it. I am determined to carry on with my life to the best of my ability.

In April 2005 I return to the MND clinic for a routine follow up. For the first time I am seen by the palliative care doctor who is based at the Calvary Hospital. "Will you be staying in Sydney or returning to New Zealand?" she asks. I know that she is really asking if I will be requiring palliative care in Sydney and will I die in Australia? I try to answer her, but again I find that I just can't utter the words without crying. The words just won't come out of my mouth. She hands me some paper and I write I'll go back to New Zealand *when I can't manage here by myself.* She talks about the options for medication to help with the continuing emotional lability and suggests that I should see a psychiatrist. *I'm fine when I'm not trying to tell people what is wrong with me,* I write.

I make an appointment to see a female psychiatrist at a private clinic in the city. The clinic is about a 20 minute walk from the central station, the appointment will last about one and a half hours and with the time involved travelling to and from the clinic I will be away from home (and work) for most of the afternoon. Then the day before I am due to attend the appointment I receive a phone call from the clinic. "The doctor you are supposed to see tomorrow is sick and then she is going away. We need to rearrange your appointment" she says. I am already concerned about the amount of time that I have taken off work to attend medical appointments. I have advised my boss that I would be attending a medical appointment on the Tuesday afternoon and we have planned our workload accordingly. "You could see a different female psychiatrist on 26 May" the lady says. "I'll be working in Auckland that day" I reply. "Is it possible to see someone at the Kogarah clinic?" I ask. She tells me the name of a doctor I could see there. He is an Indian male. "I would like to see a female doctor" I reply. I really do not want to see a male psychiatrist, let alone one from a different cultural background. I just don't feel that such a psychiatrist could relate to my social situation or understand the intense grief that I feel regarding my illness and its prognosis.

Speaking on the phone to someone I don't know is hard enough at the best of times, let alone when I am starting to feel that I am being forced into a situation that I am not going to be happy with. "What about an appointment in June?" I ask. "When?" she asks. "The month of JUNE!" I reply. Again she can't understand what I am saying. By now I am becoming upset and will not be able to say anything else without crying so I end the phone call by hanging up. I seem to be doomed. Why are things so difficult?

I am a little concerned that the lady from the psychiatric clinic has not called me back either to arrange another appointment or at least to see if I am OK. I was clearly getting upset when I ended the call with her. For all she knows I could have gone and jumped off the balcony. Surely the staff of a psychiatric clinic has a duty of care to their clients.

A couple of days later a letter from the psychiatric clinic arrives in the mail. Surprisingly the letter has the return address of the clinic on the back of the envelope! I am sure that this is against the privacy regulations. Australia has stricter privacy regulations than New Zealand has and I know that in New Zealand health instuitions are not allowed to identify the sender on mail that is sent out to patients. It's a case of not alerting other members of the household to the fact that the recipient of the mail is attending a specific health facility. For example how would a daughter explain to her parents that she was attending a sexual health clinic or in my case a psychiatric clinic? Fortunately I live alone so no harm was done.

I decide to ask the palliative care doctor what I should do with regard to arranging another appointment. As I am having increasing difficulty speaking on the telephone, I send an email via the nurse coordinator at the clinic to the palliative care doctor.

In my email I write

> I am asking your advice. The appointment that I had with the psychiatrist for this afternoon (Tuesday) was cancelled because she is sick and then she is going away – they didn't say for how long but gave the impression that I will not be able to see her. The other options for a psychiatric consultation that I was offered were not acceptable to me. One possible appointment (26 May) that was offered at the city clinic was while I will be away in New Zealand working. The other option was to see an Indian male psychiatrist at the Kogarah clinic. I don't really want to see a man; particularly one from another culture who I don't think will be able to empathise with my social situation.
>
> However, knowing now that the psychiatric clinic has rooms at the St George Private Hospital, I would prefer to see someone locally if I need to. I am conscious of the amount of time that I

> have taken off work to attend medical appointments and I am keen to keep this to a minimum while I can.
>
> I feel that part of my distress is caused by grief related to my condition. I am determined to carry on with my work for as long as I can and get distressed thinking of what the future holds in terms of missed opportunities.
>
> What do you suggest?

A week or so passes. The palliative care doctor contacts me and arranges to visit me at home. She comes to my apartment and discusses psychiatric referral. She arranges for me to be seen by a male psychiatrist at the city clinic. Reluctantly I accept as this seems to be the only option available. She assures me that this doctor will empathise with my circumstances. We discuss changing my medication from Amitriptyline to another drug. This new antidepressant does not have the added benefit of causing a dry mouth although she mentions an additional drug that I can take to dry the secretions. She leaves me a prescription and we discuss the timeframe for changing over to the new drug. I need to have a week of 'washout' off the Amitriptyline before starting the new drug. I agree to make the change after I return from a work trip to Auckland.

"I am glad that I have seen you in your home," she says as she is leaving. She can see that I am managing very well and there is no cause for concern.

A friend from New Zealand is coming to stay with me and I think that this will be a good time to stop the Amitriptyline as I will have company if I have any unpleasant withdrawal symptoms.

As it happens my friend postpones her visit. Also I feel so much happier and more confident after my week in Auckland that I decide not to switch over to the new drug. I remember when I started on the Amitriptyline there was an instant improvement in my speech and I have been sleeping so much better. I am reluctant to take a chance that my speech will deteriorate without the mouth drying effect of the amitriptyline and I do need to sleep well at night to be able to carry out my busy schedule. Knowing that I will be very busy in the next few months I am not prepared to make any changes that might jeopardise my ability to function in my job.

I wonder if some sort of counselling might help. I've worked so hard to get where I am. I have been very successful in starting a new career and now, for reasons that I can't control, it's all going to end. **I am just so pissed off about it.** I just can't shake the intense disappointment that I don't have a long term future in a job that is perfect for me. One of the requirements in the job description for a clinical research associate is 'excellent verbal communication skills' so now I feel quite inadequate because I can't express myself fluently. I am certainly not ready to accept the possibility of imminent death and I get upset thinking about it. I am determined, however, to carry on with my life and work to the best of my ability for as long as I can.

Eventually in mid-June the time comes for me to attend the appointment with the psychiatrist. I get up early and catch the 7:30 train to Central Station and then walk the 20 minutes to the psychiatrist's rooms for my 8:15 appointment. When I arrive the office is in darkness so I wander off and return 10 minutes later. The receptionist is a young man with dark hair in dreadlocks tied at the back in a pony tail. I pass my referral letter to him and sit down. Glancing up I watch him open the letter and toss the envelope into the waste bin. As my referral letter had been written by the palliative care doctor I had written a note on the front of the envelope asking for a copy of the clinic letter to be sent to my neurologist at the motor neurone clinic.

"I just saw you put the envelope in the bin" I say. "Please get it out, a letter needs to be sent to my neurologist and his name and address are on the front of the envelope." He retrieves the envelope and attaches it to the referral letter. This reinforces the negative feelings that I already have about this clinic and I very nearly get up there and then and walk out.

Something inside my head says *You have waited this long to see the psychiatrist, don't give up now.* So I sit back fuming and wait.

As it happens the psychiatrist turns out to be a very nice man and he is easy to talk to. He asks the right questions and struggling through the tears I manage to convince him that I am not depressed. I am very motivated; I enjoy my work and I have lots of things that I am looking forward to. I don't feel that life is hopeless; I am sleeping and eating well. Apart from having MND life is very good! He agrees with me that I have had some unfortunate experiences during my initial medical appointments last year and he is going to arrange for some grief counselling for me at Calvary Hospital. I am happy with this arrangement as Calvary is only a five minute drive from where I live. It will be easy to get to the appointments and will not impact on my work.

Three weeks pass and I have not heard from anyone with regard to an appointment for grief counselling. During these three weeks I have been working out of Sydney for several days each week but I am available by email and on mobile phone. Each time I return home I anxiously check the letter box, but nothing arrives from the clinic. For me time and quality of life is precious. I don't know how much time I have left. How much longer will I be able to work and remain living in Sydney? When will I have to return to New Zealand? This is the source of much of my grief. So I send an email to the psychiatrist:

> I am following up on my consultation with you on 21 June 2005. At the consultation you suggested that I should be able to receive grief counselling at Calvary Hospital in Kogarah. The letter dated May 23 that I received from your clinic confirming the date of my June 21 appointment with you mentioned that a letter summarising the outcome of the consultation with you would be sent to me and my referring doctor. I have not received a copy of the summary of our consultation or information on who I should contact for grief counselling at Calvary Hospital.
>
> My current work schedule means that I am out of Sydney for several days each week so I am anxious to arrange an appointment that will fit in with my work commitments.

Thanks and kind regards,
Barbara Williams

I receive a prompt reply from the psychiatrist:

Apologies for this

I don't routinely send copies of letters to referring doctors to clients as well although some of the clinicians here do.

I sent a letter to Dr. X some weeks ago, as well as to your neurologist.

I don't formally have links with Calvary Hospital, and intended that Dr. X would be able to organise this for you.

I will email her in the next few days to clarify whether this can be arranged and if so who may be the contact person for this.

Later that day a second email arrives from the psychiatrist:

I've emailed Dr. X and am awaiting a reply.

So it seems that the delay (or maybe misunderstanding) is on the part of Dr X, the palliative care doctor. The palliative care doctor had been slow to respond to my earlier question regarding psychiatric appointment. I know that she has a young baby but patients requiring the services of a palliative care team for whatever medical condition should, by the very nature of the service, be able to receive prompt attention.

Days pass and still there is no response from Dr. X.

In an email to Margie about my next MND clinic appointment I also mention:

When I saw the psychiatrist he suggested that I would benefit from seeing the grief counsellor at Calvary Hospital. He emailed Dr. X on (I think it was Monday this week) to remind her to organise this. I have not heard anything from her yet. I am anxious to organise this because as I said earlier there are very few week days that I am in Sydney.

On Monday the next week there is a message on my phone from Dr. X explaining that she has been away for a week. She would like to know more details about the sort of counselling that I would like. I reply by email:

> Thanks for your call. The psychiatrist thought that I would benefit from some grief counselling. He agreed with my feeling that I am not depressed. I am very motivated and have a very busy work schedule, I don't think that the immediate future is hopeless and I have lots of short term plans.
>
> I get very upset thinking of the longer term in terms of missed opportunities and the impact of MND on my ability to do what I want to do. This becomes apparent when I am forced to discuss my symptoms with the medical people who are looking after my clinical care. I no longer have a problem talking about my condition to friends and colleagues once they have gotten over the initial shock of the diagnosis.
> In fact I have just spent 3 hours in our Sydney office talking to my boss. I maintained a conversation with him for 3 hours and apart from a husky and somewhat monotone voice I had no trouble speaking - if anything my speech is better than it has been earlier in the year.
>
> So in summary - I would appreciate the opportunity to have some sort of grief counselling.

In a follow up phone call the palliative care doctor mentions that Calvary Hospital has bereavement counselling (for bereaved family members) but not the type of grief counselling that I am seeking. However she will make enquiries and get back to me.

I am really surprised that a hospital providing palliative care and hospice services has no regular counselling service of the type that I am seeking. Surely counselling is an integral part of care for people who are diagnosed with a terminal illness, whether it is a disease where death is imminent or one like MND which is incurable and the end result will be death sooner or later. It's almost as if the attitude is "OK you have a terminal illness, we'll look after you physically and make your passing as comfortable as we can. We will comfort and counsel your family. But for you – you are not supposed to get upset about it."

Some time later in the book *Rowing Without Oars* written by Swedish journalist Ulla-Carin Lindquist, I read that the motor neurone disease team caring for her includes a counsellor who is considered to be the most important member of the team.[3] This reinforces my feeling that counselling is needed.

A little further on in Ulla-Carin's book she talks about how Hippocrates in his wisdom felt that they would seldom cure, often ease, but always comfort. Ulla-Carin contrasts this with today's medical care which she feels can usually ease and cure but seems to lack the time to comfort.[3]

Yes. What about comfort? What about it? Have the pressures of everyday life, fighting the traffic to get to work, juggling home and health professional responsibilities – the reality of contemporary clinical care-taken priority over basic human needs?

I'm not being self righteous over this. In my days of providing clinical care I have been as guilty as the next person in focusing on clinical care and neglecting the comforting aspect of care.

Like most people, I have always taken my life and good health for granted. Even now I get up in the morning and get on with my day, taking for granted everything that I am able to do. I don't sit around feeling sorry for myself. My life is too busy to do otherwise.

Several weeks pass. I have had no feedback from the palliative care doctor regarding grief counselling. In an earlier phone conversation she mentioned something like "Maybe your GP will have to arrange this." However she did say that she would get back to me. I have not been happy with the GP that I have seen twice in Sydney. At the first consultation he referred me to an ENT surgeon, whom he described as 'the best in Sydney.' The outcome of consultations with the surgeon has been described earlier. In April 2005 I visited the same GP to get a flu vaccination. In recent years I have had several flu vaccinations in New Zealand. The procedure is always the same. Firstly a questionnaire regarding allergies and any previous reactions to the vaccine is completed, the injection is given and then you have to wait for 20 minutes in case you have an allergic reaction to the vaccination. In this case the GP said "OK I can do that for you." He grabbed my arm, injected the vaccination and said "That will be 12 dollars." This GP did not ask if I had had previous flu vaccinations, any allergic reactions and he did not ask me to wait for 20 minutes to see if I had an allergic reaction.

The area where I live in Sydney has a diverse ethnic mix. This ethnic mix is reflected in the ethnic mix of the GPs that practise in this area. Sometime ago Margie at the MND clinic had given me the names of two female doctors in this area whom she said were good. I would particularly like to see a female GP with the same ethnic background as myself. One of these doctors has an English sounding name and the other has a Middle Eastern sounding name.

In July 2005 I realise that I will need repeat prescriptions for some of my medication soon and I decide to make an appointment to see the English GP. I phone the doctor's office and say "I would like to make an appointment to see the doctor as a new patient." The receptionist says "I'm sorry, the doctor is not taking new patients at the moment" "I need to see a goo….a goo….." I am trying to say that I need to see a good doctor but the words just will not come out of my mouth. I hang up in frustration. Why is everything so difficult?

Instead I decide to see my Auckland GP while I am in Auckland a few weeks later. I have not seen him since before my diagnosis of MND one year ago. I check that he has received copies of letters from the MND clinic outlining my care and I mention that my next clinic appointment is in mid September. "They seem to be looking after you well in Australia" he says.

Later in August I receive a letter advising me of my next appointment at the MND clinic. In the letter I am asked to 'bring a referral letter from my local doctor.' I decide to renew my efforts to see the doctor I tried to see in July who was not taking new patients.

I write a letter to the doctor:

> Some weeks ago I phoned your receptionist to make an appointment to see you as a new patient and I was told that you are not taking on any new patients at the moment.
>
> The reason that I am writing to you is to ask if you would consider seeing me as a new patient. I moved to Australia 2 years ago from New Zealand. Since arriving in Australia I have been diagnosed with Motor Neurone disease.
>
> I was referred to a neurologist after a protracted and somewhat unsatisfactory series of medical consultations here in Sydney. My MND is now being managed by the Multidisciplinary MND service at the Prince of Wales Hospital. I mentioned to Margie, the MND nurse coordinator, that I was not happy with the GP who I had seen in Kogarah and asked her if she could suggest a suitable GP who I could see. She gave me your name..........................
>
> My immediate need is for a GP referral letter for my ongoing specialist care. If you are unable to see me, is it possible for you to suggest an alternative GP who I could see?

I post the letter and the next day I get a phone call from the doctor's receptionist. "The doctor has received your letter and is able to see you" she says and suggests a date for an appointment. "The only days that I can come are tomorrow morning or Friday September 16," I reply. I have great difficulty in saying the word sixteen and it sounds something like "sueeessseen." "I'm sorry I can't understand you." The more I try to say "16" the worse it sounds. I try to say "fourteen, fifteen, sixteen" but she still can't understand me. Then she realises that I want to come on a Friday. "September 2nd?" she asks. "No." September 9?" "No." September 16?" "Yes," I reply. Finally she is able to give me a date and time for the appointment. It is just SO FRUSTRATING!

I've wandered a bit from the subject of grief. From day to day I just get on with my work and make future plans both for work and social activities. However, my feeling of loss and sadness is still there under the surface. At the local library one day I come across a section of self help books. Many of the books have titles to do with coping with grief or loss. Scanning the introduction and contents of the books, however, it is clear that the purpose of these books is to provide support for bereaved relatives rather than the person who has the terminal illness.

Later I search on the internet for 'grief and the patient.' Most papers relate to care of the bereaved relative or to terminal care. However, I find a paper published in the American Family Physician entitled *Identifying and managing preparatory grief and depression at the end of life*. This paper acknowledges that almost all dying patients will experience grief and it is important to distinguish between preparatory grief and depression. The authors, Periyakoil and Hallenbeck, note that it is normal for people with a terminal illness to grieve for things such as missed opportunities and changes in self-image and that their grief should be facilitated and supported.[4]

Periyakoil and Hallenbeck distinguish between grief and depression. Grief, they say, often comes in waves and it is OK to cry. Grieving patients maintain a normal self-image and a sense of hope. They look forward to special occasions and visits from friends and family.[4] Why, I wonder (again), did the health professionals caring for me think that it's not OK for me to cry and want me to see a psychiatrist to be treated for depression???? I AM NOT DEPRESSED!! Don't they realise that I am grieving?

1 Joan Didon. (2005) *The Year of Magical Thinking*. Knopf: New York. ISBN 1-4000-4314-X

2 Weiner J (2004). *His Brother's Keeper*. Harper Collins: New York. ISBN 0-06-001007-X

3 Lindquist Ulla-Carin. (2005). Rowing without oars. John Murray: London. ISBN 071956686-X

4 Periyakoil V.S., Hallenbeck J. (2002). *Identifying and managing preparatory grief and depression at the end of life*. American Family Physician; 65: (5) 883-90.

6

Living and working with Motor Neurone Disease

From the time of my initial diagnosis I resolve to carry on living and working in Sydney for as long as I can. I remember telling my friend Barbara that I had MND and also saying that I still have lots of good times to come. In a way I feel fortunate that my mobility has not been affected. I can live independently even though my speech and swallowing are slowly deteriorating. I continue to go to the gym every day that I am at home in Sydney, walking on the treadmill and using the exercise bike for 40 minutes. It's not so easy to get to the gym when I am away on work trips. I make up for it by walking briskly through the airport terminal corridors, racing past other able bodied people, and in some cities I am able to walk from the hotel to the hospital.

Fortunately I work from home and this makes it easy to eat the correct food when I need to and to take my medication at the right time. My employer has been very supportive. Currently I am the sole CRA in the company and he could easily have had doubts my ability to cope with the workload and concerns that I would let him down. My work schedule has been busier than that of many younger and healthier people. During my first year with the company I made 21 work trips to New Zealand (often to several NZ cities in the same trip), nine to Melbourne and one to Adelaide. Travelling is not demanding because I am able to take taxis to and from the airports. I arrive early so I don't have to rush. I can check in at the Qantas Club counter and work or read in the Qantas Club while I'm waiting for my plane. Staying in hotels when I'm away from home makes it easy too. I have not taken one day off as sick leave and I have easily made up for all the time required for my medical appointments by working in the early mornings, evenings, and weekends.

As time goes on, I am heartened by the messages of support that I receive from friends and colleagues. In late March 2005 even though I am not a Catholic, I take inspiration from the Pope's public suffering and his determination to carry on to the end. I feel that if he can do it so can I. However, at the same time I wonder how fair this is on my employer, the various sites that I visit in the course of my work and in time friends and family if I become dependant on them for care.

At my first visit to the Motor Neurone clinic I weigh 53.3 kgs and at 151 cms I have a BMI of 24. Thus my weight is within the accepted range. Weight loss is one of the predictors of survival and I learn that if my weight drops by 10% which is roughly 5kgs, insertion of a percutaneous endoscopic gastrostomy (PEG) feeding tube will be necessary. Knowing that this procedure will eventually be necessary, I make a concerted effort to stick to the high protein, high energy diet that has been advised. I enjoy eating my favourite foods. I also start to eat desserts. I haven't regularly eaten desserts for years, being conscious that if I do I will put on too much weight. Consequently my weight see-saws a bit while I try to get things right.

While on the South American cruise with my mother I enjoy the wonderful food on the ship. Most mornings I have a bowl of oatmeal, a very runny porridge compared with how I make it at home, followed by bacon and eggs or bacon and pancakes. We usually eat a buffet style lunch of meat, salad and a small dessert. Some days I have a hamburger and chips from the pool side café. The evening meal consists of five courses. I usually pass on the soup, salad and entrée, preferring to have the main course and a dessert. This is the last time that I really enjoy eating steak, even though I have to cut the meat into thin slices to be able to chew it. Eating slowly, I'm always the last person at the table to finish eating.

I realise that I have lost the muscle tone in my face, cheeks and bottom lip. The fasciculation in my tongue is easily seen. My tongue is like a bag full of jelly that is shivering. I liken it to the abnormal heart rhythms of atrial and ventricular fibrillation. No wonder I have problems speaking, eating and drinking. I can't move food about in my mouth as I chew and food tends to get stuck on the roof of my mouth or around my gums. When I chew I tend to bite the inside of my lower lip. When I drink several mouthfuls one after another, for example when I am swallowing tablets, my back teeth bite the inside of my cheeks. And of course my speech is often slurred or indistinct.

Late in March 2005 I buy a blender and start to make a conscious effort to eat soft food that is easy to chew. I am re-discovering casseroles; pork, kumera and pineapple; chicken and mushrooms; beef and mushrooms. It's been many years since I have cooked casseroles so my initial attempts are a bit of trial and error. One bonus of living alone, however, means that one casserole will last for several meals and I make good use of my freezer and microwave. I have put on a couple of kilograms since Christmas but I am not too worried about it, knowing that as my swallowing deteriorates I will lose weight. In the meantime I make the most of being able to eat things that I enjoy.

The dietician at the MND clinic gave me a brochure for "Tender Loving Cuisine," a company that delivers frozen home cooked meals to your door. It's mainly aimed at the elderly living alone. It is an ideal way for me to introduce variety into my diet and the meals are really much nicer that the frozen meals that can be bought at the supermarket and much nicer than the hospital meals. Initially I ordered the small meals but I think that that the small ones are for little old ladies who sit at home all day. I'm not quite at that stage yet, so my second order is for the larger meals.

Sometimes it's a juggling act to fit meals around my medication. To aid absorption Riluzole should be taken on an empty stomach and also food should not be eaten for one hour after taking the tablet. I want to get the maximum benefit that I can from the medication so I follow this regime rigorously. I seem to have an internal alarm clock that wakes me at about 5am whether I am in Australia or

New Zealand, and even on the cruise in South America I seemed to wake at about 5am. I take my tablet and usually go back to sleep for a couple of hours. This works most mornings. The evenings are a little trickier. I need to make sure that I don't eat anything for two hours before and one hour after taking the tablet – effectively this is 3pm to 6pm. I try to stick to this regime whether in Australia or New Zealand where the time is two hours ahead of Sydney time. To fit in with social activities I sometimes need to vary the time that I take the tablet. In August 2005 at the Cardiac Society conference in Perth where the time is two hours behind the time in Sydney I decided to take my Riluzole at 3pm (5pm Sydney time) so that I could participate in the wine and cheese poster sessions between 5pm and 6pm. This meant setting the alarm to wake up at 3am to take my morning tablet.

As my speech deteriorates, I start to have trouble making myself understood. Early in 2005 I was issued with a light-writer voice machine on loan from the NSW MND association. Firstly the machine has a dead battery so I have to send it away to Melbourne for a new battery to be installed. When the light-writer is returned I am hesitant to use it. I feel self conscious and I am reluctant to attract attention by using the machine in public. The light-writer is slow and clumsy to use and I find it quicker and easier to write what I want to say on some paper.

I can still make myself understood even though speaking for any length of time is difficult. Towards the end of April 2005 I spend a week in Melbourne training Judy, who is a new clinical research associate from an affiliated CRO based in Japan. Judy is a lovely person and I feel really awful that my voice is letting me down. Every time I try to speak to her, I cough. Living alone and working from home I don't usually need to speak much and most communication is by email. Even when I am out at hospitals, most of my time is spent alone reviewing research and clinical documentation. Now I am particularly distressed to find that I can't say what I want to when I want to and I renew efforts to tell colleagues of my problem.

Shortly after this in the beginning of May I travel to Auckland for the weekend. My granddaughter is celebrating her third birthday and we have planned a small family gathering. On the flight from Sydney to Auckland after eating a piece of chocolate that was on the dinner tray I take a mouthful of wine and I choke. I cough and cough. Fortunately I have a serviette handy and can cover my mouth. By the time I have finished coughing and spluttering the serviette is wet. On the flight from Auckland back to Sydney I choke on a chocolate mint. Again more coughing and spluttering.

Once I start to cough, often I can't stop. It's like there is a tickle in my throat that I can't shift. Sucking a cough lozenge seems to settle the cough. The cough lozenges that I have found to be the best are 'Throaties original pastilles.' The 'Throaties' that are sold in New Zealand are a brighter red colour than the ones that are sold in Australia. The Australian ones seem to create sticky mucus in my mouth. So I usually stock up on the New Zealand 'Throaties' on my trips to New Zealand. Returning to Sydney on Sunday evening after the birthday weekend I notice the customs people stop my suitcase as it goes through the agricultural X-ray. "Is this your arrival card?" the customs lady asks. "Yes" I reply. "Do you know what is in your bag?" she asks. "Yes" I answer. She opens my bag and pulls out a plastic bag of 'Throaties'. "What are these?" she asks. "They are for my cough" I reply. My voice is husky and convinces her of my need for cough lozenges.

When I travel I carry a photocopy of a letter from the Motor Neurone Disease clinic that gives details of my condition and the medication that I am taking. I have not needed to use it yet either for emergency medical assistance or to satisfy any questions that the immigration and customs people might have about my medication.

There was a questionnaire insert inside one packet of my Riluzole tablets advising of the Rilutek Care service. I responded to the questionnaire and checked the box indicating that I agreed to be contacted by the Rilutek Care coordinator. Therese, the coordinator, has contacted me from time to time to see how I am getting on. She asks me if I am having any problems with the medication, checks that I am having my liver function monitored and offers to send me any information that I need. She sends me a British information booklet on MND that is very helpful. She also sends me a 12 hour timer and a night light. The timer is useful. I have found it easiest to take my medication at 5am and 5pm. If I don't wake at 5am the timer wakes me. Then after taking my medication, I go back to sleep. At the end of the working day I am sometimes distracted and twice I have forgotten to take my medication so again the timer's alarm is a useful reminder. I guess this is one way that the pharmaceutical company can keep track of who is taking the medication and also become aware of any side effects that may occur.

Arriving at the chemist shop one Friday towards the end of May 2005 to collect a repeat of my Riluzole tablets I am dismayed to learn that the pharmacist has not been able to obtain any of the tablets from his supplier. Because the tablets are so expensive they are not kept as shelf stock and are ordered in when needed.

"I have one tablet left for tonight's dose - what can I do?" I ask. "I'll phone around and see if I can get some. I'll phone you and let you know" the pharmacist replies. Time ticks on ..... Friday afternoon is running out and I'm aware that I'm off to Auckland on Tuesday morning so I need to get the tablets by Monday at the latest. I decide to make some calls myself. First I phone Margie the MND Clinic Coordinator and leave voice messages on her phone and on her mobile. Next I phone the 1800 number for Therese the Rilutek Care Coordinator. "This is Therese the Rilutek Care Nurse Coordinator" the answer phone says. "I'm out of the office until Tuesday, please leave a message." I need to speak to someone NOW not on Tuesday so I don't leave a message.

Next I look up the pharmaceutical company on the internet and find a number for the Multiple Sclerosis (MS) Care coordinator. Knowing that MS is also a neurological condition I phone this number and get another answer phone! "My name is Barbara Williams" I say and leave my phone number and a short message about needing some Riluzole. Having worked in both clinical and pharmaceutical industry positions I have learned to keep trying all avenues till I get a result. Knowing it is Friday afternoon I am determined to get a response before the end of the day.

I phone the Drug Company's phone number. "I would like to speak to a sales rep or a marketing person for the drug Riluzole" I say. "Who do you want to speak to?" the lady asks. "Can I speak to Therese the Rilutek Care Coordinator?" I ask. "Who do you want to speak to?" "THERESE" I spell it out. Still she can't understand me so I hang up.

Back at the website I find an email address for the Multiple Sclerosis team and I send an email:

> I am a patient with MND and I am taking Riluzole.
>
> My pharmacist is NOT able to obtain a repeat of the drug which I need URGENTLY – I have one tablet left for tonight and 5 more repeats that are unable to be filled because the chemist can't obtain the tablets.
>
> I am going to NZ for work (1 week) on Tuesday, so I need the tablets URGENTLY.
>
> I have bulbar palsy and speaking is difficult – your telephone operator could not understand me. I tried to phone Therese who is the Rilutek care nurse coordinator but her answer phone says she is not available till Tuesday.
>
> Please advise me what I should do.

Friday afternoon is ticking on and there is no response. After a while I send a similar email to the company's medical information email address and then have another go at trying to contact someone via the company's telephone operator. The telephone operator at the pharmaceutical company where I used to work knew everyone and I felt sure this company's operator would know someone who could help me. "Listen to me" I say. "What are you saying?" "Just LISTEN!" I try and speak slowly and clearly. Again she can't understand what

I am saying and I give up. I end the conversation by hanging up again.

Mounting frustration only intensifies my distress and I cry uncontrollably. I am just SO FRUSTRATED with myself for not being able to speak clearly enough for the telephone operator to understand me. It's bad enough having a disease for which there is no cure, a disease that is relentlessly progressive, and having a speech impediment caused by the disease without also having supply problems with the one drug that slows the progression of the disease.

Later in the afternoon my efforts bring some results. Firstly Peta from the drug company phones. "Hello Barbara, I got your message. We do have a problem with supply and this is what we can do" she says. "On Monday we will courier a month's supply to you. Can you fax us your prescription?" she asks. "The prescription is at the chemist shop" I say and give her the chemist shop phone number. Still I have no medication for the weekend. Both the pharmacist and Peta assure me that missing a few doses is not a problem. That's not the point though – I am determined to take the medication strictly as prescribed to get the maximum benefit from it and I don't want to miss any doses. Then I receive an email from Margie, the clinic coordinator:

> I should be able to get you some today that can carry you for the weekend. After work today, I will swing by Calvary Hospital to pick it up from my office, and drop it off to you...Is this OK?

Later in the evening Margie brings me the tablets. As a former colleague once said to me "You need to stick to something like a dog with raw meat until you get a result."

On Tuesday I travel to Auckland. In the course of my work in Auckland I meet up with several former colleagues. By now they all know so I don't worry about trying to pretend that nothing is wrong and I enjoy chatting to them. While in Auckland I also attend a clinical research conference. I find that I know many of the delegates. Talking in a crowded noisy room is difficult for me and several times I wander off to a quiet area for a break. However, I manage to speak to most of the people that I know. I am heartened by their genuine expressions of support. Later I get an email:

> Just a quick note to say Hello again and it was great to see you in the weekend. You are so positive and I admire you so keep it up.

I recall the words of the respiratory specialist. In suggesting that I should stop work and return to New Zealand to the care of my family he said "You can't pretend that it's not happening." I have worked so hard to get to where I am with my career. I am passionate about my job and I would feel cheated if I had quit work. No one can predict the progression rate of MND. It is different for each person.

I have been worrying that as my speech deteriorates friends and colleagues might find it difficult to talk to me and avoid meeting me. But so far this has not been the case. On Saturday evening Kevin and I have dinner with a couple who have been good friends for many years and on Sunday I have lunch with a group of women I used to work with. I do a lot of talking over the weekend and even though my voice is croaky and sometimes I need to repeat some words, people can understand me. I feel much happier and more confident of my ability to communicate.

7
Spending time with family and friends

When I return to Sydney I realise just how good it was to spend time with family and friends over the time that I was in Auckland. I decide to make an effort to get together with family and friends whenever I can while I am still able to talk.

My friend Barbara from Christchurch finally comes over to Sydney to stay with me. She had been planning to come to Sydney during the New Zealand Queen's birthday weekend in early June but postponed the trip because she had a cold. I choose to sleep on the couch in the living area of my one bedroom apartment and Barbara sleeps in my room. This makes it easy for me to get up early in the morning to take my medication at 5am. At 7am I like to get up, turn on my computer and start work while the North Americans are still in their offices. This way Barbara can continue to sleep and I can get on with my work dealing with anything that needs an urgent response. Barbara is staying for 10 days. On about day three or four of her visit she mentions that she has a sore throat. Within a day or so this has developed into a cold. Despite my best efforts to keep clear of her germs, it is near to impossible in my small apartment.

A few days later I travel to Auckland for work, leaving Barbara in Sydney to finish her holiday. While I am in Auckland I develop a cough. I don't know if it is Barbara's cold or not but I cough and cough for days and have difficulty talking. The cough starts as a tickle in the throat and every time I breathe out the tickle makes me cough. Talking also irritates my throat and makes me cough. I can often control it with cough lozenges though towards the end of the day the cough is worse. Being with other people when I can't stop coughing is really awful. I feel dreadful and it is really anti social to be coughing so much, even if I am not infectious. When I arrive back in Sydney I'm exhausted.

I am only back in Sydney for four days when I have to travel to Christchurch for seven days followed by a day in Wellington on the way home. I had planned this trip to span a weekend so that Barbara and I could spend the weekend at the South Island resort of Hanmer Springs. We had been planning this for many months and I had been looking forward to sitting in the hot thermal pools with the surrounding winter snow. However Barbara has another cold so we cancel the weekend at Hanmer Springs.

I contact my son Dylan who is still working in Christchurch. "How would you like to come with me on the Tranz Alpine train on Sunday?" I ask. "Awesome!" is his response. The train goes over the Southern Alps via Arthur's Pass to Greymouth on the West Coast. We have a lovely relaxing day in the train even though the typical West Coast rain starts at Arthur's Pass and is constant on our westward journey to Greymouth. The rain continues until we pass through Arthur's Pass again heading east back to Christchurch. Dylan and I are both disappointed that there is no snow at Arthur's Pass.

I have dinner with Dylan a couple of times while I am in Christchurch. When I am in Wellington I also have dinner with Barbara, who, over her cold, is now in Wellington working. However, I am still plagued with the cough and find it hard to talk during these dinners. It's just so awful. I want to be able to have normal conversations over dinner but I just can't. On one occasion back in my hotel room after dinner I cough and cough and cough until I vomit.

My sister Jenni and her husband Francis plan to have a holiday in July at a resort at Palm Cove north of Cairns in Queensland. "Barb, would you like to come with us?" Jenni asks. Fortunately I am able to arrange to take a few days off work. Jenni and Francis are travelling from Auckland to Cairns via Sydney and we meet in the domestic terminal at Sydney airport and travel together on the three hour flight to Cairns.

Arriving at Palm Cove we check into the Beach Club and Spa Resort. Palm Cove is a small beachfront village between Cairns and Port Douglas. The resort is right on the beach and there are lots of small cafes and restaurants in easy walking distance along the road. The day before we arrived a storm had caused beachside erosion and flooding at the beach immediately to the south of Palm Cove. The weather is still not the best, it is windy and overcast with scattered showers and the temperature is 24-25 degrees. There is better weather in Sydney while I am away!

On Sunday morning we go for a brisk walk along the beach. The beach slopes steeply to the water's edge and walking in the soft sand I find that I have trouble keeping up with Jenni and Francis. Yet I regularly walk at a brisk rate on the treadmill at the gym in Sydney. In the evening over dinner Jenni asks "How did you feel when you found out what was wrong?" My eyes fill with tears and I can't answer. Sometime a day or so later Jenni wonders aloud "Is it better to die suddenly in a car accident or to have something like this that gives everyone time to prepare?" I can't answer, it's like asking if you would rather be deaf or blind. What a choice - you just cope the best that you can with what life brings.

Later in the week we go on a snorkelling trip to the outer Great Barrier Reef. The boat leaves from Port Douglas and it takes one and a half hours to reach the reef. The weather is still not the best, the sea is choppy, the wind is 24 knots and the underwater visibility is not ideal. However, I have always been a good and confident swimmer and I have done lots of snorkelling as a child at Hatfield's beach and more recently in the Pacific islands. Donning a wetsuit, fins, mask and snorkel I get into the water. Instead of my natural confidence in the water, I feel less buoyant than usual. Also I have trouble breathing through the snorkel; my top lip does not make a good seal around the mouthpiece of the snorkel and water seeps in. I feel very insecure and quickly get back on the boat. One of the crew suggests that I use a polystyrene floatation aid that he calls a 'noodle' and this makes all the difference. Using one hand to keep my lips closed, kicking and using the other hand, I manoeuvre through the water to the reef. Even so, I still have trouble with the waves and the current and don't stay in the water very long. I think that my arms and legs aren't as strong as they used to be and I am easily tried. At a second spot on the reef I get in the water again and manage to see lots of tropical fish and feel that it has been a good day.

The next day is sunny and we lie by the pool. "The water is lovely" Jenni says. "Come for a swim." The pool is like an artificial beach with a sandy slope into the water. I wander over the sand into the water up to my thighs. The water is cold! It takes my breath away. The gentle slope drops away suddenly to a depth of two meters and I feel that once I am in the deep water I will not be able to breathe. I feel that if the water was warmer I would be OK. It's crazy because as a kid growing up in New Zealand I spent all my summers in the water swimming. It's this awful disease, slowly taking my strength away and with it my confidence.

Later that afternoon I say goodbye to Jenni and Francis and head to Cairns airport and the return flight to Sydney. It's been a special few days with my sister.

A week later I fly to Perth to attend the 53rd Annual Scientific Meeting of the Cardiac Society of Australia and New Zealand (CSANZ). It was one year ago at the CSANZ meeting in Brisbane that colleagues from Auckland who had not seen me in the year since I left Auckland noticed a difference in my speech and asked me what was wrong. One colleague took me aside to ask what was wrong. "I wonder if you have a Bell's palsy" she said. "There's nothing wrong" I replied. However, I started to cry. I felt so stupid because I had nothing to cry about. I was elated to be in Brisbane and to be able to catch up with all my New Zealand colleagues. I was keen to tell them how much I was enjoying living in Sydney and to tell them about the new job that I had started just two weeks ago. I now know that the tears were part of the bulbar MND.

In Perth a year later people give me a hug and comment on how well I'm looking. I haven't lost weight and I do look well. Unless I open my mouth no one would know there was anything wrong. A few mention in a kindly way that just a year ago I did not know what was wrong. I meet a professor from New York whom I have not seen for three or four years. "You are looking well" she says. I assume that she has heard of my illness from a colleague and I mutter something that prompts her to ask if I have been ill. "I have ALS" I reply almost in tears. I still can't tell people without getting upset. Later as I am leaving the evening welcome reception I meet a colleague from Adelaide. "I'm going, my voice is worn out" I say assuming that she knows what is wrong. "What's happened to your voice? Have you got a Bell's palsy?" she asks. "I've got motor ….. neurone……….." my throat tightens and I can't finish the sentence. It's just so bloody awful! As I walk back to my hotel I think *Next year's meeting is in Canberra. I wonder if I will be there? Will I be confined to a wheel chair, unable to talk? Will I even be alive?*

Again I switch from being a healthy looking, well known and respected professional to a vulnerable person with a shocking incurable illness. Will this ever stop?

Saturday, day two of the conference, I meet more former colleagues. Warm friendly hugs and words of greeting. No need to mention what is wrong. One former colleague has troubles of his own. "Are you OK?" I ask. A reassuring hug, a pat on the shoulder, no need to say more.

"Barb, you have done really well, you have attended all the sessions of the conference and kept up with everyone," Mary, a colleague and friend from Auckland, says on the last day of the conference.

On Monday evening I fly back from Perth to Sydney arriving at 10:30 pm. I take a taxi from the airport to my apartment. I enter the elevator and swipe my card to gain access to my floor. Nothing happens. I swipe the card again. And again. Still nothing. I swipe again and press the basement car park level. Still nothing. I will have to walk up the stairs. I consider leaving my suitcase in the elevator and pushing the elevator button from my floor to retrieve my bags. *What if someone takes my bag?* I think. So I start to walk up six flights of stairs carrying my medium sized suitcase and my computer bag. By the third floor I am puffing. I need to stop and rest after four or five stairs. Progress is slow. Eventually I reach the sixth floor and my key opens the stairway door into the lobby. I open the door to my apartment and pull my bags inside. I'm breathless and absolutely stuffed!

On Tuesday at lunchtime I go out to post a letter. The same thing happens when I return. My swipe card will not activate the elevator. I send an email to the property company that manages my apartment.

> On my return last night at 22:30 my swipe card would not activate the elevator to take me to my apartment on 6th floor. Consequently I had to carry my suitcase up 6 flights of stairs. Today (1pm) I had the same problem and had to walk up to my apartment.
>
> PLEASE have this repaired URGENTLY. I have a respiratory condition and get breathless walking up stairs.

True to character, I try all avenues. Next I phone the property company and speak to the manager. "I'm sorry dear, I can't understand you. Can you send an email?" "I have sent an email, I'm anxious to get something done because I'm going away again," I reply. Shortly I get a reply:

> Hi Barbara,
> I will get onto this asap...
> Sorry for the inconvenience caused...

Later that afternoon I am waiting for a taxi to take me to the airport for my next work trip (Christchurch this time) and I realise that I have left my mobile phone behind. The taxi arrives. "I've left my mobile phone in my apartment. Can you please wait while I go and get it?" I ask. Yet again my swipe card will not activate the elevator and I run (or walk as fast as I can) up the six flights! It just hasn't been my day!

I travel from Christchurch to Auckland to spend the weekend with my family. Late on Friday afternoon I email the property company:

> Do you know if this is fixed yet? I have been away from Sydney working since Tuesday afternoon. I will be returning to Sydney Sunday evening and don't want to have to drag my suitcase up the stairs again?
>
> Thanks for your help.

A little later my mobile phone rings. "Can you tell me what the problem is with the elevator?" a man asks. I explain that my swipe card won't activate the elevator to stop on my floor. I'll be able to fix it on Monday" the man says. "I'm in Auckland and returning home to Sydney on Sunday evening." I reply. "I can't carry my suitcase up six flights of stairs!" I say, starting to get frustrated. I pass the phone to Kevin who explains things further. It becomes apparent that the security company has made changes to the access codes for the elevator to tighten security in the building. Kevin reads out the security numbers on my access card and the man promises to re-programme my card so that it will activate the elevator when I return home on Sunday evening.

Arriving back in Sydney my heart is in my mouth wondering whether or not my swipe card will activate the elevator. Fortunately it works and the elevator takes me swiftly to my sixth floor apartment. Things are looking up!

8

One year on - August 2005

It's the end of August 2005 and one year since I started the series of medical consultations and tests that eventually led to the diagnosis of motor neurone disease. I still find it hard to believe that I have an illness that will kill me. I am working full time and my work schedule is as busy as it ever was. I would rather be busy than sitting around feeling sorry for myself. I thrive on being busy. I still get up each morning keen to get started and eager to see what the day will bring.

In a novel that I read recently I came across a story about the 'Precious Present.' The old man wouldn't tell his grandson what the 'present' was but he said that it would bring him lasting happiness. As the child grew he received special birthday presents and he wondered if any of these were the 'Precious Present,' but he became bored with the gifts and they didn't bring him lasting happiness. When the boy became a man he married and he thought that his wife must be the 'Precious Present' but in time they split up. Then the man travelled to beautiful places but each time he wanted to look for another beautiful place and he wondered if the 'Precious Present' was ever attainable.

And so the story goes on until one day his grandfather died. As he recalled the happy times he spent with his grandfather he realised what it was that made his grandfather so at ease and content. His grandfather didn't dwell in the past because he couldn't change what had happened. He didn't live for the future, which might never come. He lived for today. The present. The here and now. *El momento - ahora.*[1]

I try not to worry too much about what the future holds.

For 12 weeks in a row I have been out of Sydney for at least two days and up to 10 days. One of those trips was my holiday at Palm Cove and another was the conference in Perth. The rest were monitoring visits to hospitals in New Zealand or Australia.

My speech has deteriorated but most people can still understand what I am saying. Someone who doesn't know me or know what is wrong with me might think that I am missing a few sheep (or roos) in the top paddock or am drunk. I stay at the same hotels and by now the staff have got to know me, although they don't know why my speech is slurred and indistinct. I phone and order room service dinners and try hard not to slur my words. It's harder with taxi drivers, particularly those for whom English is not their native language. Sometimes I have had to write the address down on paper.

One weekend in Auckland I go to a travel agent to drop off the deposit for our summer holiday. "I am here to see Rowena" I say to the receptionist in the monotone, hesitant voice that is characteristic of my current speech. "ROWENA IS ON THE PHONE" the receptionist says loudly making a telephone sign with her fingers held up to her ear. "PLEASE HAVE A SEAT AND WAIT." I realise that she thinks that I'm deaf! I don't say anything, however, I deliberately stand and move around impatiently while I am waiting.

Another day in a hotel in Christchurch I phone room service to order dinner. For dessert I ask for "banana chocolate sponge with ice cream." I have to repeat this several times before the room service person says "thank you, it will be about 20 minutes." When the meal arrives as well as the dessert I had ordered there is a brimming cup full of drinking chocolate! "What's that?" I ask. "I didn't order that!"

The following week on a flight from Auckland back to Sydney unable to open the screw cap on my bottle of wine I ask the cabin attendant "Can you open this please?" She can't open it either and passes me another bottle that she has opened. "Are you travelling on your own?" she asks. "Yes" I reply. "Do you need assistance when we arrive in Sydney? We have people who can help you." "No I'm fine" I reply.

My swallowing has also deteriorated but by modifying my diet I am still able to eat well enough to maintain my weight. I find that I am enjoying food more and more even though I often struggle to chew and swallow some of my favourite foods. I am also still able to swallow regular fluids. I struggle to drink a whole glass of wine. I get halfway through and my throat seems to get sensitive and then I choke on a mouthful. I have always enjoyed a glass (or two) of white wine in the evenings so I persevere but these days I rarely finish a whole glass. I am having a little more difficulty swallowing my tablets. I have to take two 25 mgs Amitriptyline tablets because the 50 mg tablet is too big for me to swallow now. I have also started breaking the Riluzole tablet in half to make it easier to swallow.

My respiratory muscles have probably deteriorated too. I get breathless walking up a slight incline or climbing stairs. However I can still walk briskly on the level in airports. One evening I am walking briskly out of the customs hall into the public area at Sydney Airport when I am held up by two people pushing trolleys and walking abreast completely blocking the narrow corridor. "Can you walk faster or let me past please?" I ask. They move over and let me past. On the treadmill at the gym I walk for 20 minutes at a speed between 5.5 and 6.0 Klm/hr depending on how I am feeling. This speed is 'power walking' so I'm not doing too badly.

During the last week of August I under go a repeat brain excitability test using trans magnetic stimulation. The first one conducted in early May 2005 showed that the nerve conduction in my right hand was normal. "The nerve conduction in your right hand is basically unchanged from the study we did in May," says the research fellow when the test is finished. "The Riluzole you are taking is working. We get a real buzz when people are doing well," he says.

As soon as the date of the New Zealand general election is announced I book a return trip to Auckland using my frequent flyer points. The only flights that I am able get mean that I will arrive in Auckland at midday on Saturday and return to Sydney at 1pm on Sunday. Kevin meets me at Auckland airport and we drive directly to Chelsea School and cast our votes at the polling booth where we have both voted in previous elections. In the evening we have dinner with my sister Jenni and her family and watch the election results unfold on television.

On Sunday morning I spend an hour with my mother before heading back to the airport to return to Sydney. Because of wild weather and strong cross winds in Auckland the inbound Qantas flight is diverted to Christchurch and I spend the afternoon waiting in the Qantas Club for the plane to return from Christchurch to Auckland and to be ready to fly to Sydney. Eventually after a delay of four hours I am on my way back to Sydney. I only have carry on baggage so arriving in Sydney I am off the plane and out of the airport quite quickly.

I get into a taxi for the ten minute drive to my home. "I'm going to Kogarah" I tell the taxi driver. "Where?" "Kogarah" I repeat. The taxi driver jumps out of the car and heads off to tell the taxi controller that he has a 'short trip.' I have found that Sydney taxi drivers hate short trips from the airport and the taxi drivers are invariably bad tempered and rude to me. This driver is no exception. He drives out of the airport like a maniac. "West Botany Road - President Avenue" I tell him. The speed limit on these roads is 60 km/hour but the driver drives much faster than this weaving in and out of other cars. We make a right turn into President Avenue and as we approach the traffic lights at the Princes Highway I say "Middle lane, turn right." "What?" he asks. "Turn right from the middle lane" I repeat the instructions. Suddenly the driver swerves into the left lane and starts to turn left into the Princes Highway. "No MIDDLE LANE TURN RIGHT!!" I say loudly. "FUC...." the driver swears and turns back into the middle lane. "I can't understand your English" he says. Like most Sydney taxi drivers this man is an immigrant and English is his second language. We arrive in Belgrave Street. "Stop here" I say and quickly pay the fare of $16.75. "You don't need to be rude to me and you don't need to break the speed limit either!" I say as I get out of the taxi. Of the many bad experiences that I have had in Sydney and Melbourne taxis this one rates amongst the worst. What impression do foreign visitors get of Australia when they are treated like this by taxi drivers?

Two days later I attend my next appointment at the MND clinic. I have been busy catching up on work before I leave for the hospital and I'm running late. Rushing to get to the clinic, I arrive out of breath with a dry tickle in my throat. Consequently I start coughing when I talk to the various people that I need to see. I have my trusty 'Throaties' with me and as soon as I pop one into my mouth the coughing stops.

I talk briefly to the dietician, speech therapist, physiotherapist and occupational therapist. I'm managing well and don't need to make changes in these areas. I mention to the speech therapist that I don't find the fluid thickening substance 'Thicken up' very palatable. "I agree" she says, "it makes water seem like glue. Why don't you try the sort of juices that you can get at juice bars?" I have a blender and this seems like a good idea.

The MND family support advisor is at the clinic. She gives me a small laminated card that reads:

**I have a problem with my speech,
but I can hear and understand you.**

"Thanks, I have been thinking of making myself some cards like this for a while. The other week on a flight back to Sydney the air hostess asked me if I was travelling alone and asked if I needed help when we arrived in Sydney." "She thought you were mentally retarded" the family support advisor says. "You still have some emotional lability don't you?" she adds. I don't respond to that comment. Do people expect me to be bright eyed and bushy tailed??? I think that I am doing really well. I can talk to people now without crying, but of course I'm still really pissed off that this is happening to me!!

I have a chat to the palliative care doctor and manage to answer her questions without crying. "Your speech has changed since I last saw you. It is more nasal" she says and suggests that I should be reviewed again by the respiratory physician. I mention that I have not yet been able to find any suitable counselling. "Jessie, the new social worker, knows of a good counsellor in Hurstville" she says. When I see Jessie she is unable to find the details of the counsellor in Hurstville and gives me a brochure for a counsellor in Cronulla. Cronulla is about 30 minutes away from here by car. I still think that I would like to see someone locally so that I don't spend too much time travelling to and from appointments.

I see the neurologist. "My left hand is weak but I can still write, I'm left handed. Often my left hand is much colder than my right hand." I am wondering if it is a circulatory problem or if it is just colder because the muscles are wasted but he doesn't offer any suggestions as to what is causing it. He checks my hand grips and reflexes and he asks to see my tongue to look for the fasciculation. "What's the red on your tongue?" he asks. "I've been sucking a cough lozenge" I reply. "There is a rumour going round that you have started taking Efexor" he says. "No, I wanted to keep taking Amitriptyline. My speech has been so much better when I started taking it and also I have been sleeping much better. In fact last week when I was away I realised that I only had four tablets left so I took one each night instead of two and I haven't noticed any difference." "Then why don't you stop taking it?" he asks. "No, I don't want my speech or sleeping to deteriorate" I reply. In fact that evening, a week after reducing the dose, I am troubled by pooling saliva and a cough as I am trying to go to sleep so I go back to taking 50mgs again. He gives me a new prescription for Riluzole. I have now been taking Riluzole for one year. "You are looking well. I'm impressed" he says as I am leaving.

I chat to Margie, the nurse coordinator. "I'm having trouble swallowing my tablets. The speech therapist suggested putting them in yoghurt but I have read that fatty foods impede the absorption of Riluzole. Do you have any suggestions?" I ask. We discuss various options. The tablets are very bitter if they are crushed and put into food. Other suggestions such as gravy or ice cream are fatty. "Why don't you try thickened fruit juice?" she asks. I will give it a go, when I have time to hunt around in the shops for something suitable. But then I will still have the problem of what to do when I am travelling. I won't always be able to get suitable fluids.

Then I remember that I forgot to tell the neurologist that I have been getting gastric reflux. "I've been getting a lot of reflux, although it has been better in the last few days" I say. Margie rushes off to mention it to the neurologist. "The reflux could be caused by the Riluzole" she says when she returns. "He suggests taking the Riluzole with a meal and if that doesn't help you could take Zantac or Omeprazole." As mentioned earlier I have read that to aid absorption Riluzole should be taken on an empty stomach at least two hours after and one hour before a meal. I know that the reason the deterioration of my MND symptoms has been slower than expected is thought to be because the Riluzole is working and I am not prepared to take any risks that might stop it doing so.

The following week my lung function tests are within the normal range, slightly lower than six months ago but allowing for a margin of error, my lung function is basically the same as it was six months ago.

Strangely, even though I know that I am doing better than expected, I am not particularly elated. My mind seems to be dwelling on all the things that I am having difficulty in doing or can't do.

Just a few days later in the supermarket I find a can of apricot nectar and a few rows further along in the imported specialty products shelves I find a big carton of peach nectar. I buy both and try taking my tablet Riluzole with a sip of nectar instead of water. I'm amazed! The tablet just slips down. There is no coughing, the tablet doesn't get stuck on my tongue or fly out of my mouth as I swallow. I don't even need to break it in two in order to be able to swallow it. It's so easy that I wonder why I haven't tried nectar earlier. I am still wary of taking the Riluzole with anything other than water so I have only a couple of sips of nectar followed by a glass of water. I don't want to do anything that will impair the absorption of the medication that seems to be working so well. My next challenge is to take a bottle of nectar with me on my travels. What will happen when I pass through the agricultural inspections?

A week or so later I fall over in the street. A few times recently I have caught the toe of my floppy left foot on an uneven paving stone in the street and stumbled but managed to right myself before I fell. This time I am walking along in the main shopping street in Kogarah and the next thing I know I'm falling "Ohhh……!!" escapes from my mouth as I hit the pavement. Stunned, I'm fumbling with my sunglasses that have fallen off when I feel hands grab me by the arms and help me to my feet. An elderly gentleman has helped me up. "I'm OK" I say hoping for the best and feeling rather stupid. A younger lady asks "Are you OK? Are you going somewhere?" "No I'm OK" I say and wander off across the pedestrian crossing, making my way home up Belgrave Street.

By the time I get home my left knee is throbbing. I survey my injuries. I have several broken fingernails, grazes on my left wrist, the palm of my right hand, a graze on my left cheek, scratches on my nose and a graze on my left knee. Fortunately no bones appear to be broken. Just the day before my fall I ran down the escalator to the Illawarra train line at Town Hall station because the video screen said the train was one minute away. I really MUST be more careful. I know I must, but I've always been so active and I'm used to walking fast. It's not in my nature to slow down.

The next day in response to an email from Margie asking how I am, I mention that I had a fall. Margie replies:

> The neurologist thought you had a mild foot drop. An ankle foot orthosis (AFO) would help with this, and prevent falls caused by the foot dragging. What do you think? Do you think you may be able to pop in at some time to see the physio?

I reply:

> I'm willing to consider it. I have tripped several times but been able to save myself except for yesterday.

One afternoon a few days later I arrive at the physiotherapy gym to see Nina the physiotherapist. There are several elderly patients having therapy. This brings back bad memories of my days as a student nurse, helping stroke patients learn to walk again. A younger lady is moving plastic cones, with great difficulty, from one side of the table to the other side. It dawns on me that one day soon I may be like them. *I don't want to end up like this* I think. I still can't accept it.

Nina and the orthotist watch me walk across the room a few times. Then Nina asks me to stand on my heels and take a few steps. I can't do it, my left foot just flops to the floor. The orthotist says that an ankle foot orthosis (in simple terms a plastic splint) will stop my ankle from flexing when I walk and that at this stage it will hinder my mobility rather than help it. I'm happy with this. "I'll just have to be more careful" I say.

The following morning I'm up early to fly to Christchurch. I have no problem walking and on arrival at Christchurch airport I am able to walk briskly past the other passengers and arrive well ahead of them at the immigration desk. I have dinner in the evening with Dylan; spend the following working morning at Christchurch Hospital and visit my friend Barbara and her parents at lunchtime on my way back to the airport.

My laptop computer started making clicking noises while I was in Christchurch and then finally it died. I arranged to take the computer directly to our IT guys in St Leonards when I arrived back in Sydney later in the afternoon. At Sydney airport I get into a taxi and pass the driver a piece of paper with the address written on it. The taxi driver, who is an eastern European immigrant, hops out of the taxi to ask his mate how to get to St Leonards. St Leonards is on Sydney's North Shore. We travel along the Eastern Distributor towards the Harbour Tunnel. "I need $4.50 for the toll" the driver says to me. "Haven't you got an 'E' tag?" I ask. "No" replies the driver. I tell him that I will pay the toll as part of the taxi fare with my American Express card and I say "You should have an 'E' tag. What will you do if you have to drive through the cross city tunnel?" I ask. The cross city tunnel is 'E' tag only. "I can't understand your English" the driver says so I give up. Yet again I am frustrated by a hopeless taxi driver. In Sydney there are so many toll roads that I can't see how a taxi can remain in business without an 'E' tag. Again I wonder how many foreign visitors are misled by taxi drivers.

The following morning I am up early again to travel to Auckland for a long planned family get-together. Kevin's uncle is 90 and the extended family is having a party for him. On Saturday morning we drive from Auckland to Katikati in the Bay of Plenty for the party. It's really great to see Uncle Buster who is 90 and the aunties and cousins who have come from around New Zealand, Australia and Canada for the party. Buster's wife Norma is in a wheel chair and their grandson Ben, now in his 20s, was born with cerebral palsy and is also in a wheel chair. Ben was also born with limited hearing so the family is used to people with disabilities and speech problems. Alan from Canada has industrial deafness and hearing aids but we are able to chat away and by repeating several words he understands what I'm saying. It's a lovely day and I relax and enjoy the day and don't worry about my speech.

Back in Auckland on Sunday morning I have morning tea with Robyn, a friend and former colleague, and then we go and visit Sue, another friend and former colleague. Both Robyn and Sue have teenage boys who have recently suffered spinal injuries, one a diving accident and the other a rugby scrum accident. Fortunately both boys have made a full recovery. It's a reminder, though, of how fragile life and good health is. We take so much for granted.

I return to Sydney on Sunday afternoon and on Monday drive over to the IT guys' premises to collect my laptop with its new hard drive. Fortunately the important documents were backed up on the company server and I haven't lost anything of major importance. I have lost my internet websites and I need to re-install several other programmes and get the laptop to speak (print) to the printer. It's frustrating but I'm grateful to have the laptop fixed so quickly. The majority of my work is done using the computer and I have become so reliant on communicating by email that without it I'm lost.

A month or so ago I purchased and installed on my laptop a text to speech programme called 'TextAloud'. Luckily this is backed up on a CD and I am able to re-install it. 'TextAloud' lets you listen to text and documents on your computer. There is another programme called 'Next Up Talker' that can be loaded on to a PC tablet. As my voice deteriorates I think that I will use these two programmes to communicate.

At the moment I can usually still make myself understood although sometimes people don't understand me and I get frustrated. At the butcher shop I ask for "one pork chop, no skin." The Asian lady looks puzzled and says "one leg of lamb?" "NO ONE PORK CHOP - NO SKIN" I repeat loudly and wave my card at her.

I have Motor Neurone Disease

I have a problem with my speech
But I can hear and understand you

The very next day, Sunday, I have lunch in a food hall in the city. I ask for a lemon and sugar crepe without any problem. Then I ask for a bottle of coke. "Can I have a glass please?" I ask. The Asian lady looks puzzled. "Can I have a cup?" I ask again. She offers me a straw and says that they don't have any cups. "I can't use a straw" I say. I wave my card at her and ask for the money for the drink back. It's just so frustrating. I'm trying to get on with my life as best as I can while I still can. Mostly I can get by just saying "thank you" "yes" and "no."

A day or two later I make myself some pumpkin soup. While I am filling plastic containers with the soup a container falls from my hand and orange soup splatters all over the kitchen floor.

Blast! I have known that it is only a matter of time before things start dropping from my weak left hand. Again I NEED TO BE MORE CAREFUL!

Then only a day or so later while shopping at the local supermarket I trip over a box on the floor. There were full boxes of products in all the aisles waiting to be unpacked and stacked on the shelves. Negotiating my way between shoppers, shopping trolleys and these boxes the toe of my sandal catches a box and down I go! My shopping spills out of the basket all over the floor. A lady stops to help me re-pack my basket. "Are you alright?" she asks. "Yes, I tripped over the box" I reply. "I'll tell them that these boxes are dangerous" she says. This time it was my good right foot that caught on the box. I twisted my ankle and hurt my knee but again nothing seems to be broken and I continue with my shopping.

Now I am finding that I can't walk as fast as I have been able to. I'm still going to the gym every day that I am in Sydney and walking for 20 minutes on the treadmill but whereas I used to be able to walk at 6kmh now I start off at 5.5kmh and sometimes after 10 minutes need to slow down to 5kmh. Then I spend 20 minutes on the exercycle.

A former colleague and friend (another Robyn) from Nelson is passing through Sydney and I have dinner with Robyn, her sister and a friend of Robyn's from Sydney. We have a lovely meal at a restaurant outside on the quay beside the Opera House. It's a warm spring evening and we enjoy the magnificent views of the Sydney harbour, the ferries and the dinner cruise boats coming and going from Circular Quay and the lights in the city buildings. My swallowing is not the best though, and I'm not able do justice to the lovely wine or the meal.

Robyn reminds me that I have been promising to visit Nelson and tells me that I should do so while I am well enough to enjoy it. Racing off to catch the train home to Kogarah I promise to come and see her soon. The very next week I am due to be in Christchurch for work. Luckily I'm able to arrange my work trip for Thursday and Friday and I am able to book plane tickets to fly to

Nelson on Saturday morning and return to Christchurch on Sunday in time to catch the last plane back to Sydney on Sunday evening.

In Christchurch I have dinner with Dylan. There are two elderly ladies dining at the next table. As they get up to leave one lady stops at our table and says to Dylan "I've been listening to your mother talking to you and she sounds just like my daughter, she's deaf too." Earlier in the day when I checked into the hotel I think that the man at the desk also thought that I was deaf. I don't get embarrassed about the way I speak – there isn't anything that I can do about it. I'm more concerned that I can convince people that I am a competent professional person travelling for business reasons and I am not mentally retarded.

The following evening I have dinner in a restaurant by myself. I order my meal by pointing to what I want on the menu. "Can I have a glass of coke?" I ask. "What do you want?" the young waiter asks "Coca Cola" I say. "I'm sorry, I'm French. I don't understand" he says. "I'll get someone." Off he goes and comes back with a lady. "What do you want?" she asks. "Coke" I say. "I can't understand" she says and hands me some paper and a pen. By then I have got my card out of my handbag and show her. I feel absolutely bereft and have a hard job stopping the tears. Here I am, a respected professional away from home on a business trip and yet I can no longer ask for a simple thing such as a drink in a restaurant.

The next morning in the hotel, having learnt my lesson, I write on a piece of paper:

I would like to arrange a late check out, I will need to work in my room and send emails in the afternoon.

"That's OK, you can stay till 12 MD" the lady says. "I'd like to stay till three or four" I say holding up three and then four fingers. "That will cost an extra $40" she says. "That's OK" I reply. In comparison a relatively painless transaction.

I spend a quiet Friday evening with my friend Barbara and on Saturday morning Barbara drives me to the airport to go to Nelson.

Robyn meets me at Nelson airport and we set out. We visit the markets in the centre of town. We have morning tea with Robyn's sister who has made the most delicious bacon and avocado muffins – straight out of the oven and they are superb. I choke on a piece of onion in the muffin that has lodged in my throat. Luckily my cough reflex is still OK and I regurgitate the onion along with a mouthful of muffin - disgusting and a bloody nuisance. MND is such an anti-social illness but fortunately they understand. We have lunch at a café on the wharf at Mapua and then Robyn and her husband drop me off at the home of my friends Chris and Nick.

Later in the evening we all go to Robyn's house for dinner. Another friend and former colleague is also there and we all have a lovely evening. I'm only sorry I can't do justice to the meal and enjoy more of the wine! It's a bugger! I get part way through eating and drinking and then can't swallow any more. The muscles involved in swallowing just stop working. Even though my deteriorating speech means that I can't participate fully in the conversation I have a wonderful evening. I haven't laughed so much for a long time. None of us wants the evening to end and it's about midnight when we leave.

I have a quiet Sunday morning with Chris and Nick before catching the plane back to Christchurch in the afternoon and the evening flight back to Sydney. It's been a very special weekend.

Back in Sydney I visit my GP. I park in the street almost outside the surgery and go inside. There are several people waiting and I sit down to wait my turn. A little while later there is a sound of metal scraping against metal.... then silence...then a crash, the wall of the surgery shakes and there is a sound of breaking glass. Another lady and I get up and open the door onto the street. A car driven by an elderly gentleman has mounted the pavement and ploughed into the outside wall and glass window of the surgery. My first thought is that he has died at the wheel and driven off the road. But he moves and looks stunned so I think maybe he has had a stroke. Then the doctor comes out of her consulting room to look at the man so I go back inside and sit down. Someone comes into the surgery and mentions that the elderly gentleman says that his foot got stuck under the accelerator causing him to drive off the road. I wonder how this can happen and at the same time I think it's fortunate that so far it's only my left foot that is weak and with my automatic car I only need to use my right foot to drive. Next someone comes in asking whose car is parked outside because a parked car has been hit. I rush outside thinking that it's my car but it's the car parked in front of mine that's been damaged. What a lucky escape! I go back inside and sit down again, a little shaken by the events.

When it's my turn, I enter the consulting rooms and hand the doctor a typed note explaining what I need. A day or two later at the library I hand the librarian a typed note asking to borrow some books for an extended period while I am away out of Sydney. At the Deli I hand the shop assistant a hand written note for a thick slice of short bacon (for my homemade pumpkin soup). It makes communication so much easier - why didn't I start doing this earlier?

Sometimes, though, I need to use the telephone to communicate. Since being in Australia I have continued to use my New Zealand Visa card. The card is due to expire at the end of November 2005. I remember two years ago that I had to make a special arrangement to have the new card couriered to me in Sydney, so I phone the NZ Visa number for use by people overseas. Unfortunately the toll free 0800 number does not work when calling from overseas so I am paying for the call. A very nice young man answers after the second ring; I'm impressed that I have not been put on hold. "I'm living in Sydney and my New Zealand Visa card is due to expire at the end of November" I say. "I would like to arrange to have a new card sent to me." I give him the card number and answer some questions about recent transactions. "I'm sorry" he says "from the answers you have given I am not able to verify that you are who you say you are." As the conversation goes on I am having increasing difficulty speaking. My voice sounds like a nervous little old lady. "I'll be in Auckland next week" I say. He suggests that I go into an Auckland branch of the bank with ID and organise to have the card delivered to me while I am in Auckland. I agree to do this but by the end of the conversation it's all I can do to say "good bye" without crying. It has been distressing having to maintain a conversation for so long, knowing that the person at the other end of the phone is possibly thinking that I being dishonest in trying to obtain the Visa card.

Using my typed note strategy I go to the bank in Newmarket on my way to Auckland City Hospital. The lady is a bit taken aback at first when I hand her the note but soon she understands what I want. She takes me into an office and phones the Visa people and arranges for my new card to be couriered to my home in Birkenhead. Luckily it arrives while I am still in Auckland and all is well.

By December 2005 my work is so busy that I am away from home every week travelling to Melbourne, Brisbane, Hamilton, Auckland and Perth. I don't have major problems communicating with work colleagues. If they can't catch a word or two that I am saying, I write it down. At a start-up meeting in Melbourne for a new clinical trial I give a PowerPoint presentation using text to speech dialogue embedded in the slides. This works well and in the following couple of weeks I give training presentations using PowerPoint with embedded text to speech dialogue at hospitals in Brisbane and Fremantle.

I write my destination on a piece of paper to show to taxi drivers. However, in two hotels when I phone to order a room service meal the person on the other end of the phone says "I'm sorry, I can't understand you." The more I try to say what I want the worse my voice gets and I end up by hanging up the phone and crying uncontrollably, a combination of the pseudo bulbar effect and intense frustration. On the first occasion I eventually give up and go out and buy a Subway roll. On the second occasion a couple of days later they kindly send someone up to my room with a menu and I point to what I want. I feel awful about it. It's just so hopeless not being able to say what you want to.

1 Santa Montefiore. (2001) *Meet me Under the Ombu Tree* pp.189-191. Hodder and Stoughton. London. ISBN 0 340 77109 7

9

Christmas 2005 and the holidays

I fly from Sydney to Auckland on Christmas Eve. I have used my frequent flyer points to upgrade to business class, a good decision because the plane is full of families travelling to Auckland for Christmas. I manage to indicate my meal choice by pointing to the item on the menu. The wind is behind us and it is a fairly fast flight across the Tasman, however this means that I miss out on purchasing the duty free sun screen I had wanted. There was no advantage being in business class as the cabin attendant spent all his time doing duty free purchases for people in the economy cabin! On arrival in Auckland Kevin meets me at the airport and we go home to get organised for the following day.

We spend Christmas Day at my brother Gavin's house. There are about 30 people there from extended families. I don't talk very much and at times need to write things down. Over the next few days I visit friends and get ready for our holiday.

My original plan for Christmas was to spend a white Christmas preferably somewhere in the UK or Europe. Over the years I have attended training meetings in various places in the Northern Hemisphere in December or January and have been caught up in the exciting pre or post traditional winter Christmas atmosphere. One year I was in New York during the first week of December and, unable to get closer, I stood on the steps of St Patrick's Cathedral during the lighting of the lights on the Christmas Tree in Rockefeller Square. The following day I stood by the tree, entranced, watching the ice skaters in the rink below the tree. The Christmas decorations in the streets and big department stores, the roasting chestnuts and bell ringers on street corners along with the intense cold air temperature created a magic atmosphere.

By searching on the internet I found a small hotel in the Scottish Highlands that had three day packages for Christmas Eve, Christmas Day and Boxing Day. Another place I would like to visit in winter is Rothenburg in Germany. I visited the medieval walled town several years ago when I was in Munich for a meeting. At the time thought it would be lovely to come back in December for the annual Christmas market. We needed to book early for both places and not knowing whether or not I would be well enough to make the trip I was hesitant to make the commitment. In the end we settled on what seemed to be a safer option, a Pacific cruise.

On December 30 Kevin and I fly to Papeete to embark on a 10 day cruise round the islands of French Polynesia. Some years ago I spent an unplanned 24 hours in Papeete when returning from a meeting in Europe. I was on an overnight flight from Los Angeles to Auckland when in the middle of the night the United Airlines plane made an unplanned stop in Papeete because of a fuel leakage. It was 24 hours before the plane was repaired and we continued our journey to Auckland. As a business class passenger I had been accommodated in the Meridian Hotel and was enchanted by the spectacular mystical views of nearby Moorea. I always wanted to return.

The first island that we visit on the cruise is Moorea. The ship anchors in the lagoon and we go ashore on the ship's tender. On a bus tour around the island we drive up one of the lofty peaks to Le Belvedere lookout with the promise of sensational island and lagoon views. No mystical views though, it is raining and all we can see is the surrounding mist-shrouded tropical rain forest which is alive with mosquitoes! The lively commentary by the bus driver, a Tahitian man of Swiss and Tahitian descent, has us all laughing despite the rain.

I have a sense of déjà vu as I realise that our ship is almost identical to the one that my mother and I were on in January last year on our

South American cruise. Kevin and I are in cabin number 4008 and last year Mum and I were in cabin number 4010 – right next door but on a different ship. The passengers on the *Tahitian Princess* are a mixture of New Zealanders, Australians and North Americans, about a third of each, with a few other nationalities as well.

We have been allocated a table for the first dinner service at 6:30 pm. This suits us very well as we don't want to be up too late in the evenings. We are seated with the same four people every night. One couple are from Wellington. The other couple celebrate their 50th wedding anniversary on New Year's Day. Originally French, they moved from Paris to Australia 30 years ago. They are a really lovely couple and have many interesting stories to tell. We all enjoy each other's company at dinner and it is just such a pity that I can't join in the conversations. I find it hard to eat quickly enough and end up not finishing my meals so that I am not holding everyone up for the next course. I am quite disappointed that I struggle to drink my wine; it catches in the back of my throat as I swallow and I have fits of coughing. Eventually after a few nights, I give up and miss out on sampling some lovely wines.

It's New Year's Eve as we sail out of the Moreea lagoon. Kevin and I are both tired and we go to bed early thinking that the ship's horn at midnight will wake us. In Auckland in recent years the fireworks at the top of the Sky Tower wake me and I get up and watch the display from the window of the family room. On the ship I sleep right through 12 midnight and when I wake up on New Year's Day we are in the Tuamotu atolls north east of the Society Islands. The day is spent cruising (no stops) through the Tuamotu atolls, the largest archipelagos in Polynesia. As the ship passes by each atoll we can see the low lying islands fringed with palm trees, waves breaking on the reef, the white sand of the lagoon beaches and turquoise waters of the lagoon. It's lovely – just like the postcards. The following day we are cruising at sea heading further northeast to the Marquesas Islands.

The Marquesas Islands, 1400 kilometers northeast of Tahiti near the equator, are said to be the most isolated (furthest away from continental land) in the world. We arrive at the island of Nuku Hiva and it is raining as the ship anchors in a bay. The volcanic Marquesas Islands rise out of the ocean to lofty peaks and have no protective coral reef. We go ashore in the ship's tender. We take the free Le Truck bus (a real truck with a closed in seating area at the back - wooden seats and no windows) to the village and back again to the jetty. We don't even get off; it's too wet to walk around. It's an eerie feeling to arrive at such an isolated island with a small population; it's like another world and we are intruders.

We have more luck the following day on Hiva Oa which is the island where Gauguin lived. The rain has stopped, the sky is blue and the sun is shining as we go ashore in the ship's tender. Boarding Le Truck we travel along a winding road lined with frangipani, hibiscus and other flowering trees to the cemetery where Gauguin and Jacques Brel are buried. Then we walk down the hill to the Gauguin museum which is a highlight of the trip. There are certified copies (not originals) of many of Gauguin's paintings on display and, in contrast to other local buildings, it is really well maintained and on a par with other art galleries. Then we walk along the road to the town domain where there is a market and cultural dance show.

We have another day at sea heading back to the Taumotu atolls and the following morning the ship sails into the lagoon at Rangiora. This is the second largest atoll in the world and from the ship anchored inside the lagoon we can't see the far side of the lagoon - it is over the horizon! Going ashore in the ship's tender we walk a little way along the shore, put on our reef shoes and swim in the lagoon. The water is just lovely; we relax in the tepid water soaking up the beauty of our surroundings. A little further along the beach is a hotel with bures on poles out over the lagoon. This is paradise! I wander along a track past palm trees and houses and no more than 100 or so yards away I come to the ocean, although I couldn't see the ocean from where we were swimming in the lagoon. The atoll is all very low lying, it's beautiful, but I wouldn't like to be here in a cyclone.

Our next stop is Raiatea in the Society Islands. This island has the second largest population in French Polynesia with 10,000 people. It is the only port other than Papeete where the ship is able to tie up at the wharf. At all the other places we have to go ashore in the ship's tender. They say that Raiatea is where the first Polynesians were and from here they went to Hawaii and New Zealand. In the evening we go over to a small motu in the lagoon for an island feast. The food is cooked in the island equivalent of a Hangi. When the Hangi is opened the first thing out is a live centipede which is promptly squashed with the spade. Several local children perform Polynesian dances and then a teenage boy does a Haka. To our amusement the Haka is the New Zealand All Blacks' Haka *Kamate Kamate*. Kevin and I laugh. The Americans think it is authentic. At the end of the show we make our way back to the jetty and the boat that will take us back to the wharf and our ship. We get into the boat and the outboard motor starts up. Nothing happens, we don't move. The tide has gone out and our boat is stuck in the sand! After several attempts to re-float it we are transferred to another one and are on our way.

Sailing overnight we cruise into the Bora Bora lagoon early the next morning. Ahead are the spectacular trademark peaks of Bora Bora, the water looks lovely and palm trees line the shore. It's magical and I think that Bora Bora is my favourite island. It is Sunday and the local church is packed – all the women are wearing white dresses and hats just like the Pacific Island women do in Auckland and the sound of singing drifts out through the open doors and windows of the church. We wander around the local black pearl and other tourist shops. After lunch on the ship we go ashore again in the tender and transfer to a glass bottom boat. Out in the lagoon we see tropical fish swimming amongst the coral on the reef. I'm reminded of my snorkelling trip on the Great Barrier Reef in Queensland. "The coral is prettier in the Great Barrier Reef" I say to Kevin but he struggles to understand what I have said. The boat goes out to the edge of the reef and we can see the drop off to the deep dark ocean.

As the ship is sailing back to Papeete we have a farewell dinner. The galley has prepared a special dessert, Baked Alaska! The waiters parade around the dining room with the flaming desserts held high. I have no trouble eating this dessert and it is gone all too quickly. When seconds are offered I am quick to say "Yes please!" Everyone laughs! Roger, seizing the moment, jumps up takes a photo of me tucking into my second helping. In Papeete we enjoy a day in the sun at the Intercontinental Hotel with several of our fellow passengers before an early morning flight back to Auckland. In Auckland I change planes and continue to Sydney, back to reality, back to work.

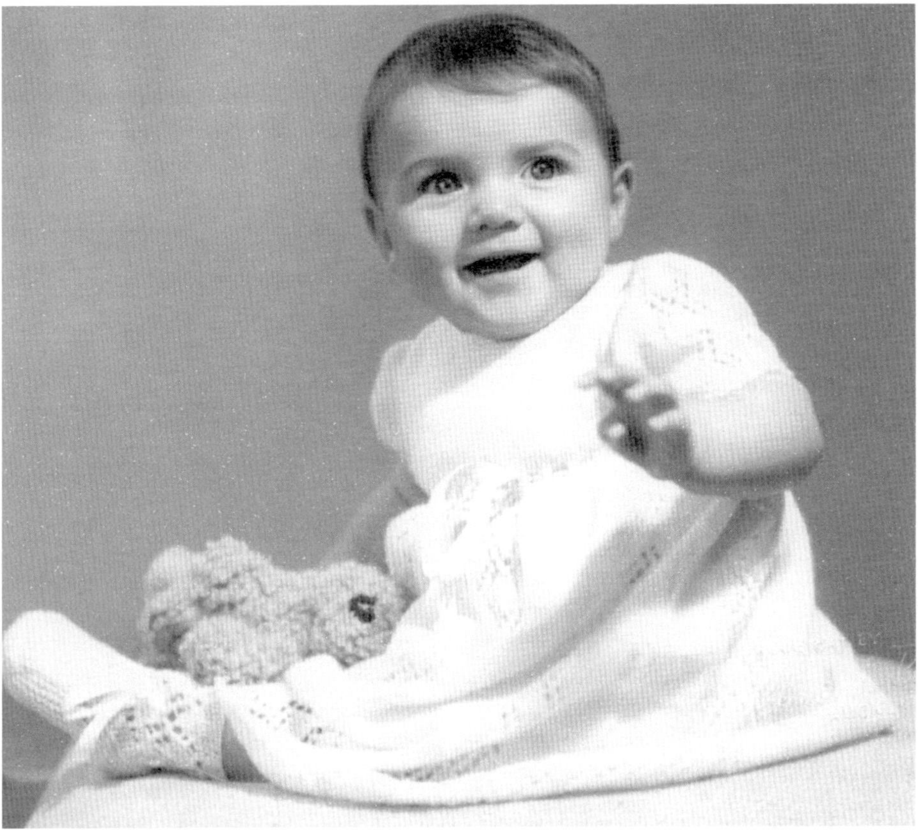

Above: *Baby Barbara.*

Below: *I'm about three years old and my sister Jenni (the blonde) is about two.*

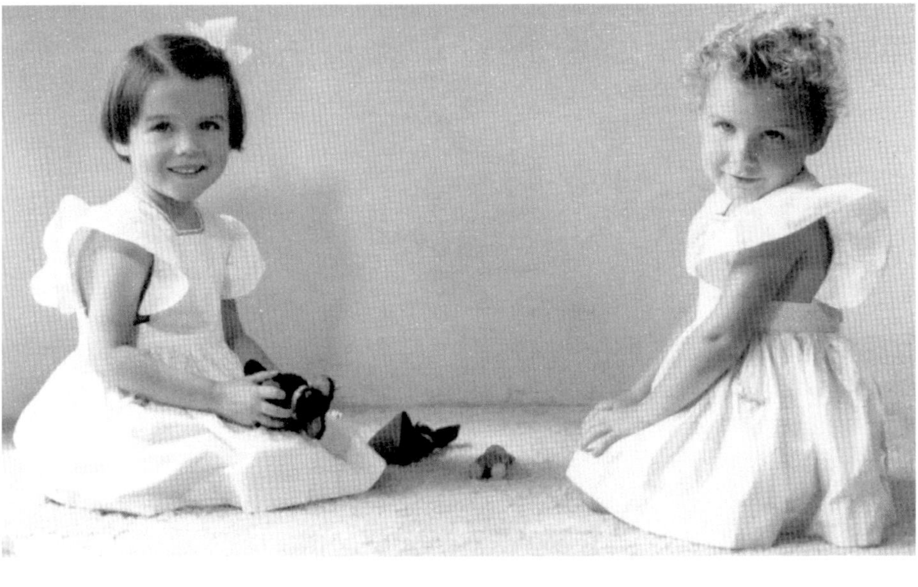

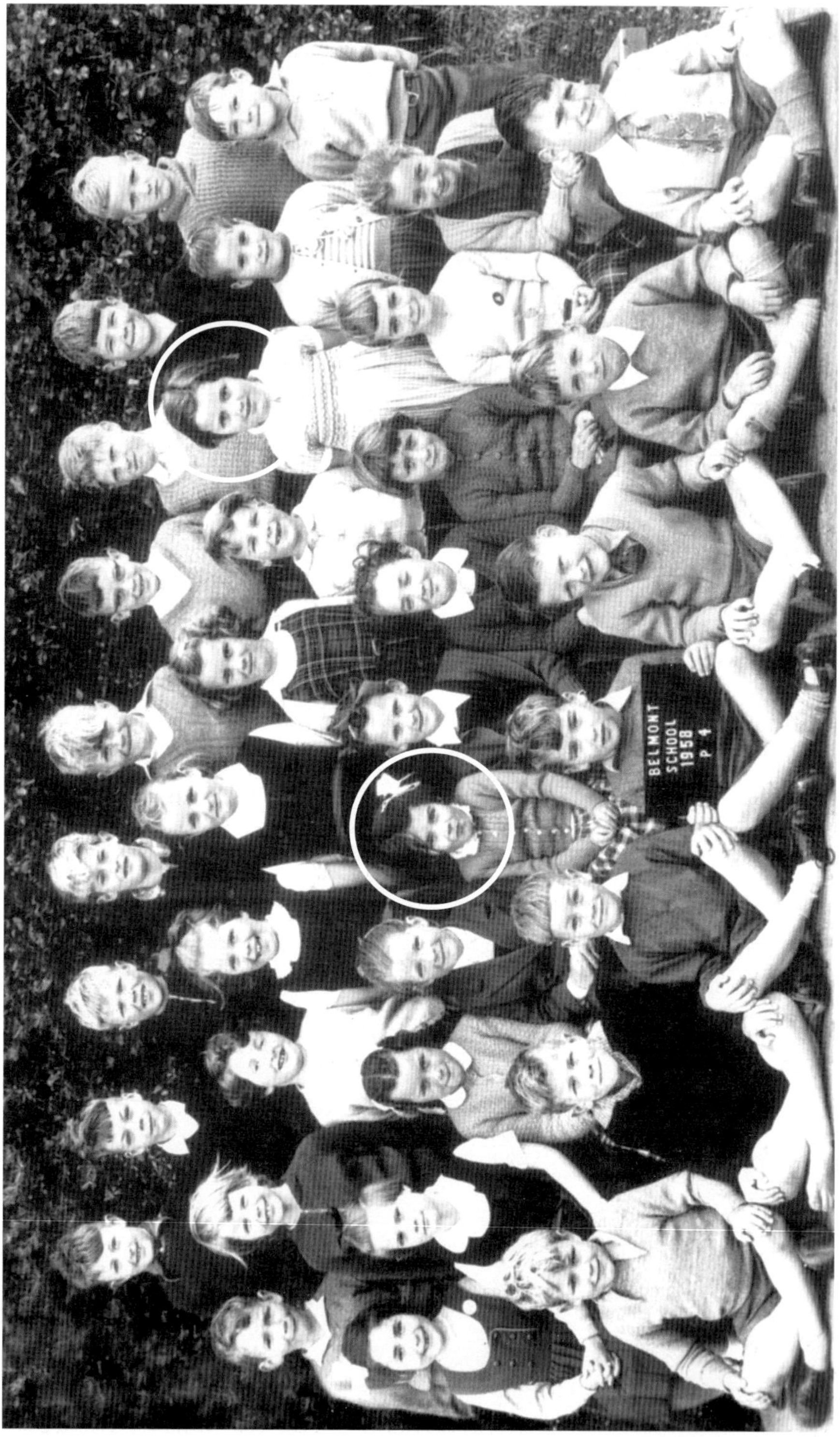

Above: *Class photo primer four Belmont Primary School. Little Barbara (me) in the second row and Big Barbara (my friend) in the third row.*

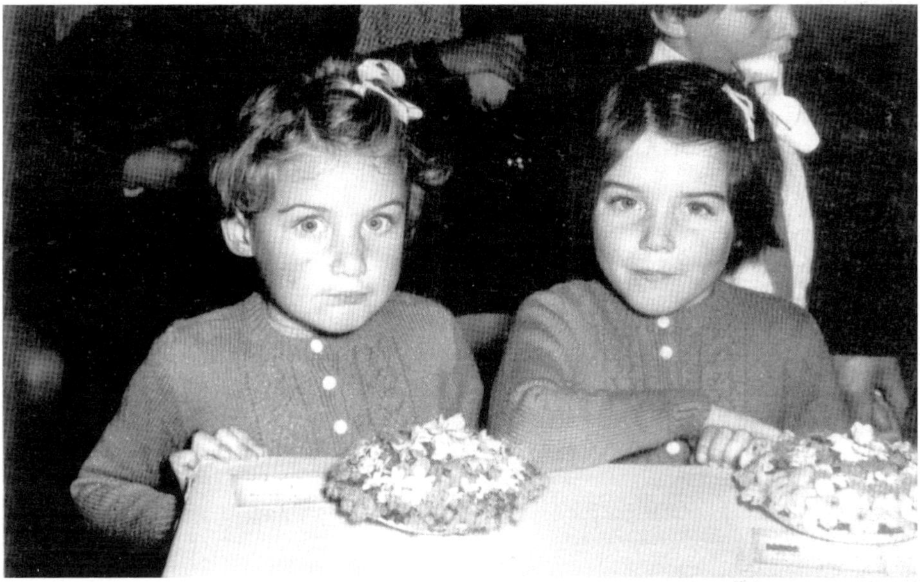

Above: *Jenni and me aged about 5 and 6 with our sand posies at the local flower show in Devonport.*

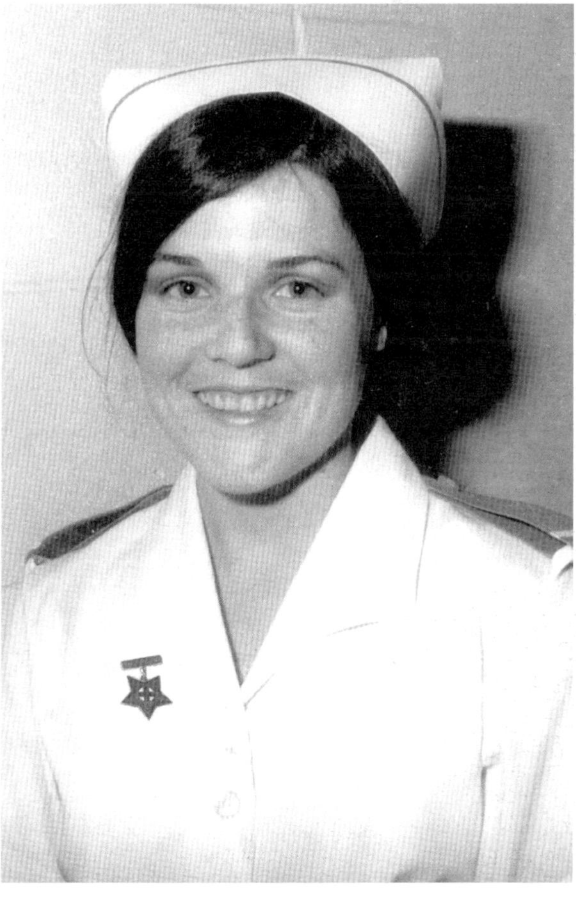

Right: *Graduating NZ Registered General and Obstetric Nurse (NZRGON); Wellington Public Hospital, June 1972.*

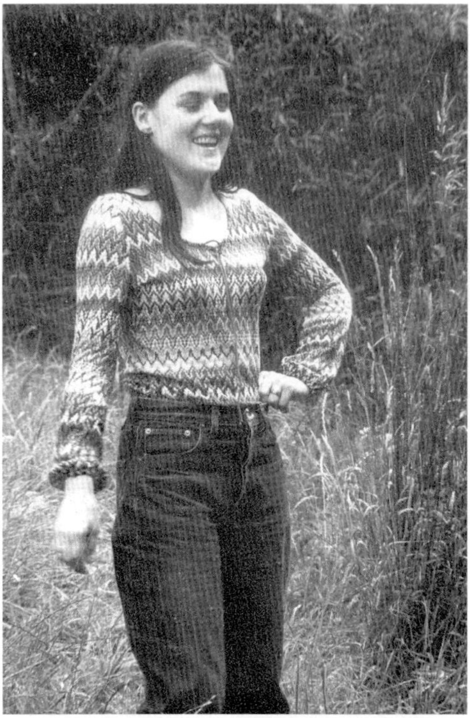

Left: *At the Wellington Polytech Design School picnic; Whiteman's Valley, 1971.*

Below: *Kevin and I on our wedding day; June 1972.*

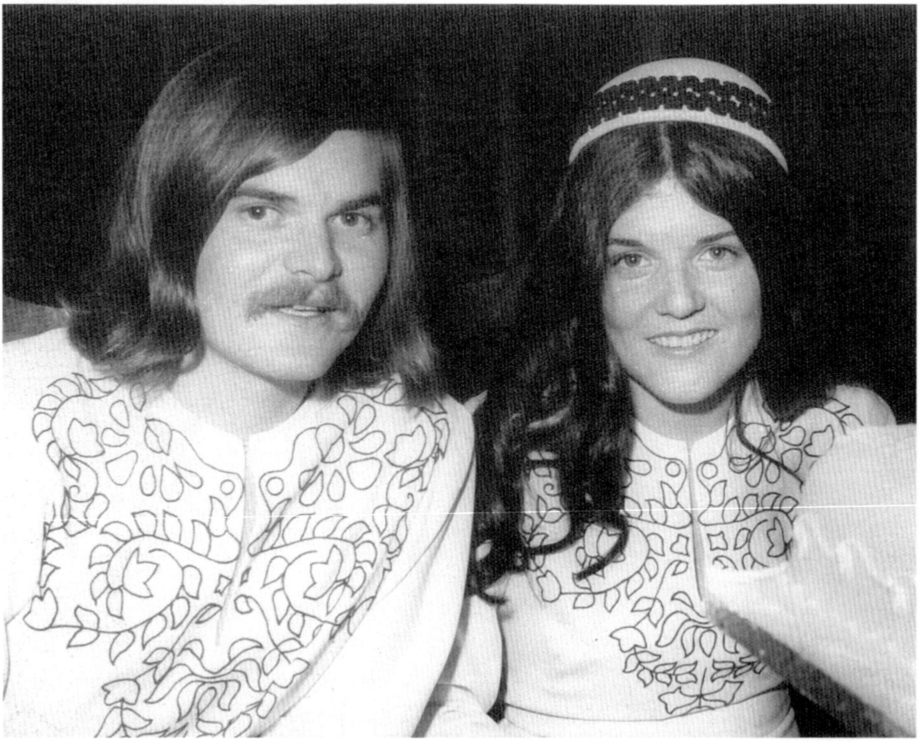

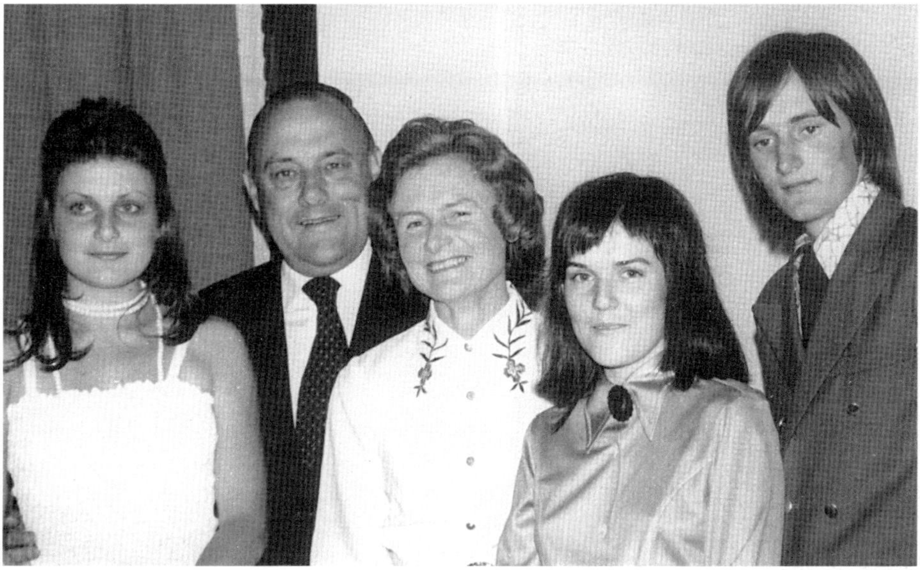

Above: *1972 with Mum and Dad, Jenni and Gavin.*

Below: *With Mum and Dad at a Family Christmas lunch.*

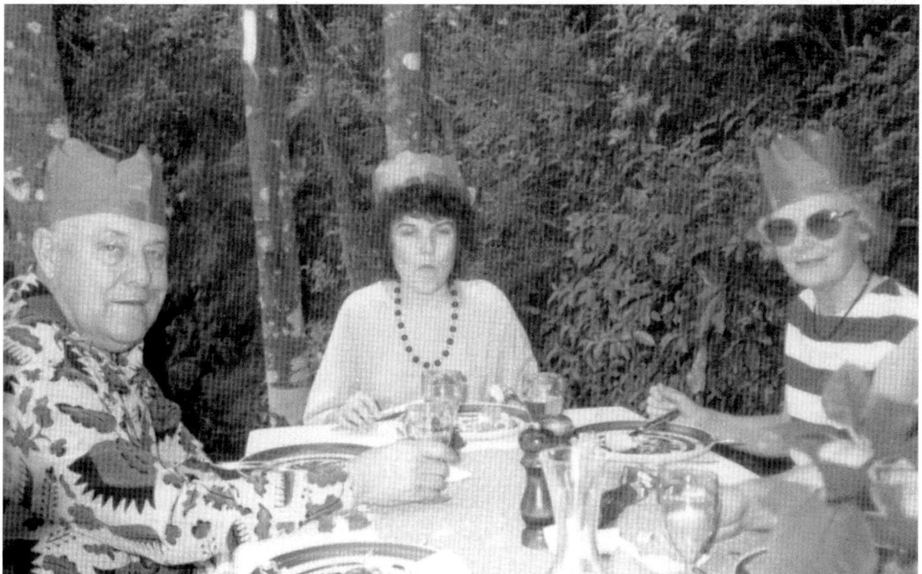

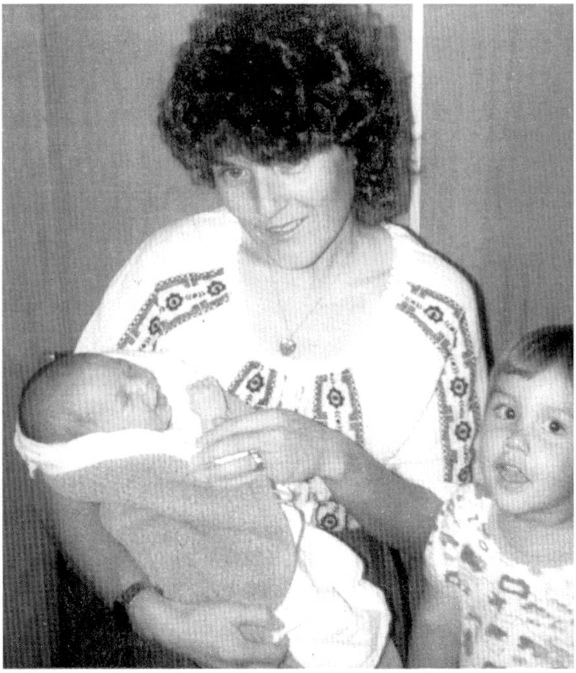

Above: *With Baby Emma and Dylan aged two.*

Below: *1983: With Mum and Dad, Dylan and Baby Emma on the garden steps at Vogel House, Lower Hutt, Wellington.*

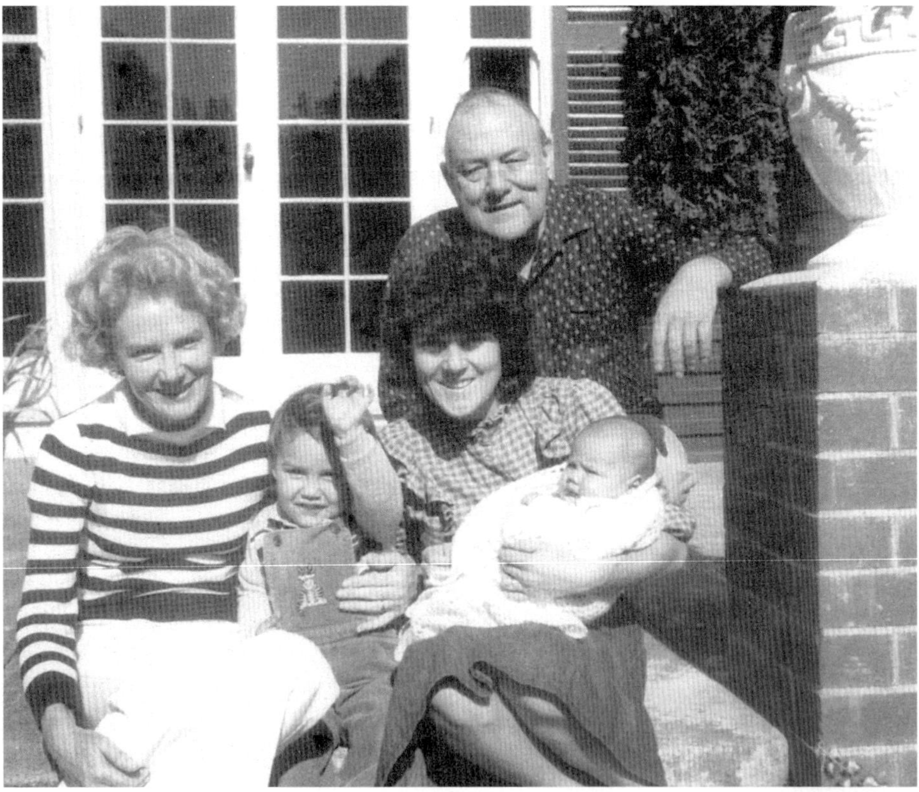

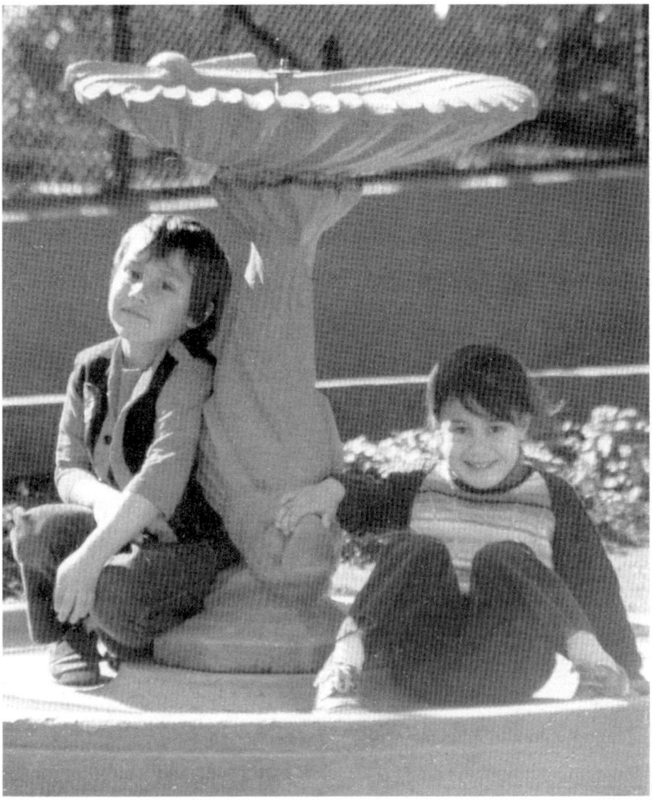

Above: *Dylan and Emma at the Auckland Zoo.*

Below: *Emma and Dylan growing up. Dylan aged 15 and aged 16, Emma at her first ball.*

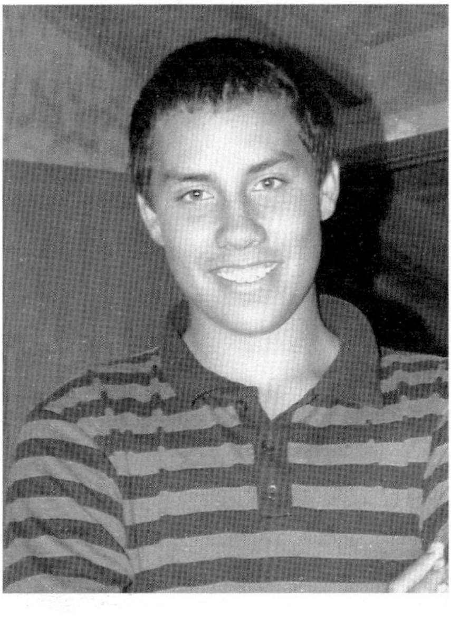

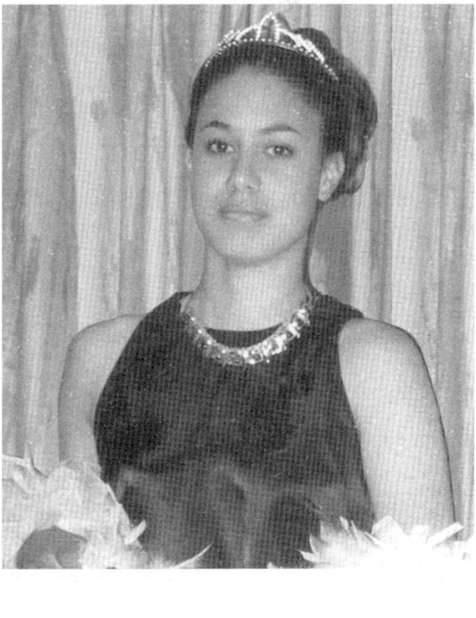

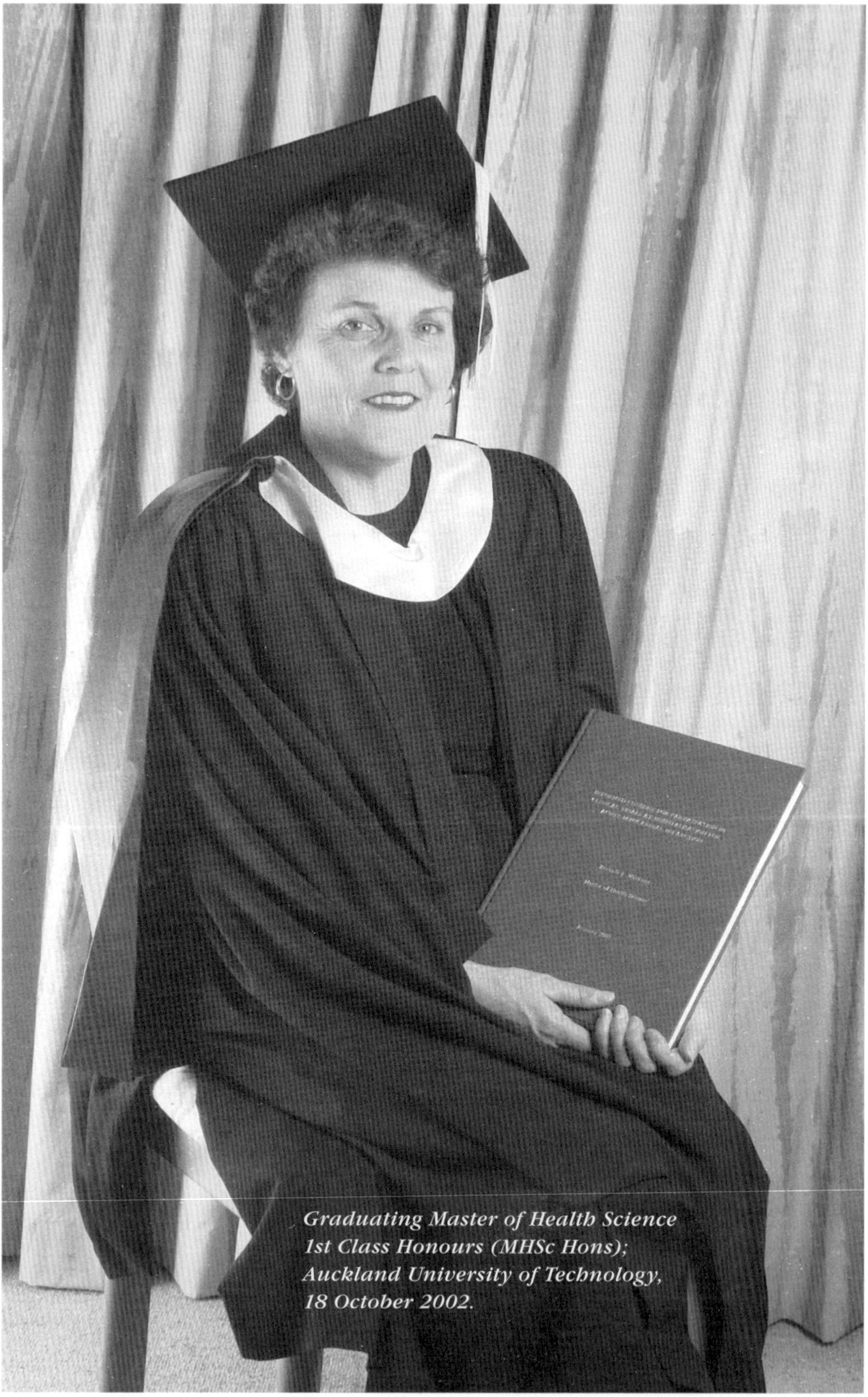

Graduating Master of Health Science 1st Class Honours (MHSc Hons); Auckland University of Technology, 18 October 2002.

10

Early 2006 - I've lost my voice

Back at work in January 2006 I resume my hectic schedule. I have a quick trip to Brisbane followed by 10 days based in Christchurch with monitoring visits to hospitals in Christchurch, Wellington and Dunedin.

I have dinner with Dylan twice. The first time I haven't brought a pen and paper with me and he has trouble understanding some of the things I'm saying. The second time with pen and paper communication is much easier. Dylan is moving back to Auckland at the end of February. I will miss our dinners together in Christchurch which we have both enjoyed.

Barbara and I finally get to spend a weekend together in Hanmer Springs. Our planned weekend there last winter was postponed because Barbara had a cold. The alpine village of Hanmer Springs 90 minutes drive from Christchurch is magical in the winter. Barbara and I went there one winter when Dylan and Emma were young. We skied at two of the local ski fields and afterwards soothed our aches and pains in the thermal pools with snow lying around on the ground. I find that the same magic isn't there in the summer but we have a relaxing weekend and enjoy the pools and the cafes and restaurants

One evening in Christchurch I have a drink (or try to drink) with two study coordinators whom I have known for many years, having met them at various meetings. It is nice to catch up with them, not that I can say much though - more writing things down. I buy the drinks, going to the bar with a hand written list. As soon as I see the glass for the coke I ask Do you have a glass with straight sides? I have trouble drinking from a glass that flares outwards because my lips, lacking muscle tone, don't seal properly and liquid spills onto my clothes. I need to drink from a glass with straight sides. The girl shows me the glasses that they have and the nearest is a wine glass for my coke. Well, more coke goes on my trousers than down my throat and in the end I give up. I've started travelling with my own glass but didn't take it to the bar; I should have!

During the course of my work people who haven't seen me since before Christmas ask me how I am getting on. I respond saying "I'm OK, but my speech is getting worse." One doctor asks me if am going to keep working. Trying to say "I will for as long as I can" I start to cry and I write for as long as I can. To reassure him I also write I'm OK.

I really am OK mentally and I'm physically OK within the limits of my physical problems. Eating and drinking is getting harder. When I am eating with other people I don't finish my meal because I am so slow that I feel as though I am holding them up. I feel much more comfortable eating by myself in my own time.

I spend four days of the next week in Melbourne visiting four different hospitals. Jo who is one of our CRAs is also in Melbourne that week working on different projects. One evening we plan to meet up with Julie who works with a Melbourne company that we have links with. I arrange to meet up with Jo at her hotel, the *Holiday Inn* which is at the opposite end of the CBD from where I am staying. I decide to walk to the there thinking that it will take about 30 minutes. It's a hot afternoon and I start off walking at a good pace, but it's further than I thought and I gradually get slower and slower and 45 minutes later I'm relieved to reach the *Holiday Inn* and sink down gratefully into an armchair in the air-conditioned lobby. No sooner have I sat down than I receive a text message from Jo asking if I have arrived. I reply and within minutes Jo meets me in the lobby. There is some confusion about where we are supposed to meet Julie and Jo suggests that we walk up the road to a bar where she thinks Julie might be waiting. The last thing I want to do is to start walking again but off we go with me struggling to keep up.

Julie is not there and we walk back to the *Holiday Inn* and wait. Eventually Julie calls me on my mobile to see where we are and I hand the phone to Jo who speaks to her. We jump in a taxi and head off to a bistro several blocks up the road. We have a lovely dinner, and I contribute to the conversation by writing things down. The next day I send an email to Julie telling her how much we enjoyed the evening and she replies:

> You are doing an incredibly gutsy job and good for you, you are a real inspiration.

A few days later I send an email to a person in the USA we will be working with. In the course of my introduction I mention:

> I also need to tell you that one year ago I was diagnosed with motor neurone disease (known in the US as ALS or Lou Gehrig's disease). My voice has been affected and I have difficulty speaking on the phone so communication by email is best for me.

I'm heartened by the response:

> Great to hear from you! Yesterday I spoke with Julie who had nothing but wonderful things to say about you. I will enjoy working with you. I am sorry to hear about your disease. I am all too familiar with it, unfortunately - but I am very comfortable with email and given our time zone differences I think it works beautifully!

In fact I have received similar responses from most of the people who I have dealings with in the USA, Europe and elsewhere. For a teleconference I email the person in the USA:

> We are on line with "instant messaging" any comments/ responses that I want to make during our call I'll send to Jo and she will be my "voice".

And after the call he responds:

> Not a problem at all, I think it worked out perfectly. Not a concern here at all. Thank you for calling in and for your time. I appreciate your hard work already.

I am so lucky to be able to continue to work and travel without too many problems.

A week or so later I'm in Perth and instead of staying at my usual hotel in the Perth CBD, thinking that I will save on taxi fares I decide to stay at the slightly more expensive *Esplanade Hotel* in Fremantle which is within walking distance of the Fremantle Hospital. I arrive in my room and try to log on to the internet using the hotel's broadband connection. In most hotels it's a simple matter of connecting up via the internet cable and clicking on the 'accept' icon and the fee is automatically charged to your room account. In my room at the *Esplanade* I find a notice 'to activate broadband internet access phone reception.' So for me who can't be understood on the telephone, I have to hike back along miles of corridors with a note in my hand asking for internet access. Then a bit later wanting a room service meal I have another hike along the corridors with another note to the bar asking for a room service meal. An hour or so later when my meal hasn't arrived another hike to the reception desk with another note asking them to chase up my meal. This time the note starts off *I've lost my voice...* and the grey-haired Scottish man behind the desk says "Oh you poor dear." I laugh!

Back in my room I reflect on the difference between the reaction of people when I show them my note *I have trouble speaking, but I can hear you* and the response from the Scottish man. Most people can relate to losing your voice and the implication is that I can speak or I have been able to speak. Whereas my note *I have trouble speaking* leaves people wondering if perhaps I have never been able to speak associating this with possible mental retardation.

Back home in Sydney I make myself a new notice:

I have lost my voice
I can still hear you

As time goes on I'm surprised at how much better I feel letting people know that I have 'lost my voice' rather than 'I have trouble talking.'

Quite unexpectedly one Friday night in March Kevin phones me to say that my friend Barbara's mother has died suddenly. I'd had an email from Barbara a couple of days earlier saying that there had been a complication following her mother's knee replacement but she was now improving. When I was in Christchurch in January Barbara had mentioned that her mother Betty needed to have a knee replacement operation. Betty had doubts about having the surgery and I assured Barbara that things would be OK as apart from her age (83) she was no more of a surgical risk than any other 80 year old. Betty had a clean bill of health from a pre-op cardiac evaluation and the surgery went ahead as planned. Unfortunately she had a series of post operative complications and despite initial improvements she died. Her death was totally unexpected. Barbara, an only child, is my oldest friend, we started school together as five year olds and Betty thought of me as another daughter.

I make hasty plans to travel to Christchurch. The earliest flight that I can get from Sydney to Christchurch is on Sunday morning and I need to return to Sydney on Monday afternoon in time for my next MND clinic appointment on Tuesday morning. I only have carry on luggage and I'm through immigration quickly and arriving at the customs check where the man asks "Do you have any more baggage to collect?" "No" I answer. I'm the first passenger from my plane to arrive at the agricultural x-ray and I need to wait while the guys pull themselves away from watching the Commonwealth games on the TV and screen my luggage. Barbara and her friend Robyn meet me at the airport and there are hugs and tears all round before we get in the car and drive to Barbara's.

A little later we drop Robyn back at the airport to go home to Dunedin and Barbara and I go to the funeral home to see Betty; more tears. I have trouble getting off to sleep; the chimes on Barbara's clock keep me awake, and the last chime I remember hearing is 1am.

On Monday morning Barbara and I take her father Bob to see Betty. Bob has Alzheimer's disease and lives in a rest home. We enter the viewing room, Bob takes one look at Betty and says, "Not alive." Bob touches the wooden side of the coffin. "Nice" he says, but we are not sure how much he understands. I find that the tears are never very far away, it's that dammed pseudo bulbar effect again.

Then I'm back at Christchurch airport again in time for my 2:30pm flight back to Sydney. I hand my passport and emigration form over to the man at the customs desk. "Why have you only been here for one day?" he asks. "Death in the family" I reply. "Excellent" he says handing my passport back to me. *He didn't understand me* I think (hope).

I found the last 24 hours emotionally draining and back in Sydney I'm exhausted. Luckily I have a good night's sleep and feel much better in the morning. By 10am I'm sitting in the waiting room at the MND clinic for my six monthly check up.

The first people I see are the physio and the occupational therapist (OT). I walk into the room and sit down. The OT is new, I haven't seen her before. She runs through her check list, "Can you toilet yourself unaided?" she asks. *I've just walked into this room and sat down unaided - what does she think?* I wonder as I answer "Yes." "Do you have a separate shower at home or is it over the bath?" she asks. I write I have a separate shower, but when I'm away the shower in hotel rooms is often over the bath. "If you have difficulty using the shower over the bath when you are away we can give you a bath board to take with you when you travel" she says. Again I wonder *what??* Just imagine me fronting up at the airport check in with a bath board under my arm!

Before my hurried trip to Christchurch I had decided to spend a long weekend in Broome while I am in Perth for work. In fact I was in the process of searching the internet for a place to stay in Broome when Kevin phoned me to say that Barbara's mum had died.

For as long as I can remember I have been interested in other places and have always wanted to travel. I remember when my father was first elected to parliament and he had to fly from Auckland to Wellington each week while parliament was in session. I was only young and I wondered how a large plane could get off the ground and fly. I wondered if it was a great conspiracy, tricking people into believing planes could fly when they really didn't.

A year or two later the King and Queen of Thailand were visiting Wellington and my sister Jenni and I were to fly there to see them. I was really excited about the trip but a day or so before we were due to leave I developed pneumonia. I was sent to stay with my grandma and I still remember how dreadfully ill I felt. I remember vomiting all over the bedclothes and Nana putting a bread poultice on my chest. My brother Gavin went to Wellington in my place. I was devastated and this still rates as one of the biggest disappointments in my life.

When Queen Elizabeth II opened parliament a year or so later Mum and Dad took me to Wellington to make up for it. Shortly after that Dad became the Under Secretary for Finance and we moved to Wellington to live. We still had our bach at Hatfield's Beach on the Hibiscus Coast north of Auckland and three times each year we flew from Wellington to Auckland to stay at the bach for the school holidays. Flying in and out of Wellington airport in the NAC (National Airways Corporation, later re-named Air New Zealand) Viscount and Friendship planes of the 1960s we got used to turbulence and I have never had a fear of flying.

I had always planned to finish my nursing training and then travel. However, I met and married Kevin and we settled down in Auckland. I have always regretted not travelling when I was younger and in many ways I'm making up for it now.

Last year I read a wonderful novel *The Kimberley Sun* by Di Morrissey. The book is set in Broome and the story spans the early years of the pearling industry in Broome through to after the Japanese attack on Roebuck Bay. This sparked my interest in visiting Broome.

On Thursday I travel from Sydney to Perth. Thursday is a work day and in the afternoon in Perth I join a web/phone based training session with participants located in New Zealand, Tokyo and the Netherlands. The training goes well and I have an early night.

Friday morning I'm up early for my flight to Broome. I've used my frequent flyer points for the plane tickets and the only seat available is in business class. The Boeing 737 has three rows of business class seats and I have seat 1D. I'm lucky enough to have an empty seat beside me and as soon as the seat belt sign is turned off I shift over to the window seat and watch as the dry and barren countryside passes by below. The stewardess asks "What would you like to drink?" I show my handwritten note *Coke - no ice - I've lost my voice*. "Are you deaf?" she asks. "No" I reply. "Will your voice get better? "No." Still, I have established that I'm not handicapped or retarded.

March is still officially the hot/wet season in Broome. I'm aware of this before I plan my trip but I'm also aware that time is running out for me and I want to do things while I'm still able to. On arrival in Broome it is 32 degrees and HOT and humid but at least it's not raining. I check in to the hotel and again I show my *I've lost my voice* note. Later I go to the reception desk with a note asking for a map. I've also written *when I booked this hotel on the internet it said that you had a restaurant*. The hotel's restaurant is closed because it's the 'off' season in Broome. The girl at reception sells me a map for one dollar and says "The Black Pearl restaurant is just across the road and is open for breakfast, lunch and dinner. Have you been to Broome before?" she asks. "No." "Have a look at this brochure. The 'town tour' is really a good way to get to know Broome" she adds.

It's too hot and humid to walk anywhere so I take the town bus to China Town and wander around the pearl shops. The shops remind me of the pearl shops that Kevin and I looked at earlier this year in Bora Bora, except that here in Broome the pearls are mostly white rather than the black pearls of the Pacific Islands. The shop assistants are very friendly and try to engage me in conversation. I mutter a slurred "Hi" and keep on looking at the pearls, hoping that they don't think I'm drunk.

On Saturday afternoon I go on the 'town tour.' I show the tour driver, Scott, my *I've lost my voice* card. Getting into the bus, Scott introduces me to the other passengers. "This is Barbara, she's lost her voice so don't think she's being rude if she doesn't talk to you." As we are driving along Scott asks everyone to introduce themselves and say where they have come from. People come from Dublin, England, Melbourne and Brisbane. "And Barbara's our mystery woman" Scott says.

In Western Australia I take my Riluzole at 3pm which is 5pm in NSW, so at 3pm I quietly fish my tablet out of my handbag, get my glass out of my back pack and fill it with water. Breaking the tablet in half, I pop one piece into my mouth and swallow it, hoping like hell that it goes down first pop. It does! Second half, in the mouth, mouthful of water and swallow. Yes! It's gone down. I wipe my mouth and put my glass and water bottle back into my pack. I wonder what the other people on the bus are thinking, but I keep on looking out the window and try to act as if nothing is unusual.

A little while later we arrive at Matso's Brewery for a beer tasting. "Can you drink beer?" Scott asks. "No." "They also have ginger beer. It's got a very low alcohol content." Scott adds. "I can't swallow" I reply. "What did you say?" "I can't swallow." The lady from Brisbane overhears the conversation and says "She can't swallow." It's such a pity; on a hot humid day like this I would have loved a beer. As well as not being sure that I can swallow the beer without coughing, it's only about 30 minutes after I have taken my Riluzole. As previously mentioned I always wait at least one hour after taking Riluzole before eating or dinking so that I don't hinder the absorption of the tablet.

The tour bus is a 14 seat Mercedes Benz people mover with a 20 inch plasma screen mounted behind the driver. Throughout the tour the slides, videos and commentary present an insight into Broome and its colourful past. The last stop on the four hour tour is Cable Beach at sunset. Arriving at five minutes to six we watch the brilliant golden sun sinking into the Indian Ocean. Dead on 6pm the last glow of the golden ball sinks below the horizon. I'm reminded of the photo that I have above my desk in Sydney, a picture of the sun sinking into the Pacific Ocean taken just over a year ago while I was on the cruise ship *Insignia* off the coast of Southern Chile. I'm only sorry that I don't have a few more days in Broome to explore further.

The tour bus drops me off at my hotel. I cross the road and go into the Black Pearl restaurant for dinner. I don't have a reservation and being Saturday night the restaurant is heavily booked. The waitress remembers me from last night. "Can I sit here?" I ask, pointing to an empty table. "We only have tables outside" she says. "I want to read my book" I mutter pointing to my book. "It's too dark out there." She wanders off to check the reservations list and then says "OK." I write down the meal that I want and sit back reading my book until the meal arrives. As I'm eating the restaurant fills up with several large groups of Saturday night diners. It gets really noisy and I feel increasingly self conscious, nibbling away on my chicken.

When I'm away I find it easier and now prefer to have room service meals so that I can take my time eating. Often food is pushed to the roof of my mouth and gets stuck. My tongue can't shift it and I need to dislodge the food with my thumb. Other times a piece of food gets stuck on the back of my tongue and I need to use my finger to shift it forward so I can chew it. Not a pretty sight! You don't realise how much the tongue assists chewing and swallowing until you lose full use of it. Eventually I give up on my meal and go back to the hotel.

On Sunday I have a leisurely breakfast at the Black Pearl and then cross the road to visit the museum before going to the airport for my flight back to Perth.

Back in Perth I have a nasty fall. Walking back to the hotel after a day monitoring at Fremantle Hospital I trip on a cobblestone just across the road from the Esplanade Hotel. I fall flat on the left side my face. While I'm gingerly feeling my skull to see what damage has been done a couple of young ladies come and help me up. "Are you alright?" one lady asks. "I.... I......I..." I'm trying to say "I'm OK" but the words just won't come out of my mouth. My left shoe has fallen off, I put it back on and one of the ladies helps me across the road. "Thank you" I say and hobble in to the hotel. In my hotel room I survey my injuries. I have a big graze above my left eye but it's covered up by hair so it doesn't look too bad. I have grazes on the knuckles of both hands and a huge chunk of skin has been scraped off the palm of my left hand. Fortunately nothing seems to be broken.

I've finished my work at Fremantle Hospital a day earlier than I had planned and I decide to change my plane ticket and return to Sydney on Tuesday instead of Wednesday. For some reason the internet booking system won't let me change my ticket on line. It keeps telling me to try again later. Time is getting on and I want to obtain a ticket for the morning flight to Sydney so I write out a note and ask the concierge to phone Qantas for me. With my plane ticket changed I go to the bar with another note to order a room service meal. The waitress delivers my meal and as I am signing the bill she sees my grazed hands "Would you like some bandages for your hands?" she asks. "Yes please." The waitress returns with the duty manager and the first aid kit. Hands bandaged I eat my meal.

I'm up at 6am and off to the airport for my flight back to Sydney hoping for an uneventful week.

Back in Sydney the script for my next lot of Riluzole is in the mail box and I take it to the pharmacy. The pharmacy doesn't keep Riluzole in stock. The pharmacist says "I'll order it for you, it should be here after 2pm tomorrow." A little later the phone rings. "Hello Barbara, it's Michael from the pharmacy. I've just contacted my supplier and Riluzole is out of stock. I'll try and get some for you tomorrow," he says.

This is the second time that Riluzole has been out of stock. I send an email to Therese the Riluzole support person at Sanofi-Aventis:

> I've just had a call from my pharmacist advising me that his supplier says Riluzole is out of stock.
>
> I have enough tablets to last me till Saturday, however this is not acceptable, Your company must have a very good idea of the number of people who are taking Riluzole, through your Riluzole care programme, and supplies should be maintained.
>
> People with MND have enough issues to deal with without the added problem of their medication being unavailable.
>
> My pharmacist has always been very helpful. I have copied him on this email so that you or one of the reps may be able to assist him in obtaining supplies.

The next day Michael phones me to say that the Riluzole has arrived.

On Friday I have an appointment with an orthotist. Last year after falling twice I had been assessed by the orthotist at the Prince of Wales Hospital who felt that an AFO (ankle-foot orthosis) would hinder my mobility. However the weakness in my left foot has slowly got worse and the physiotherapist suggested that my need for an AFO should be reassessed. This time because of service cut backs in the public hospital I have to drive across town to see an orthotist in his private practice.

I have some pretty impressive scars and a black eye as evidence of my fall on Monday and the orthotist says that I do need something to counter the 'foot drop' that is causing my falls. He discusses the options and I go for the more expensive carbon fiber AFO. This is lighter than the molded plastic one. It sounds a bit like the old metal calipers with a carbon fiber rod up the side of the leg rather than a plastic strip up the back of the leg. I'm hoping it will give me more mobility.

I have a quiet weekend catching up on work and housework that has mounted up while I have been away. As I'm walking slowly home pushing my small shopping trundler several people who are walking faster pass me. It was only a few months ago that I confidently raced past all the slow coaches at the airport. Now I am painfully aware of how slowly I am walking.

On Monday afternoon I have a repeat barium swallow. I really think I know the outcome before I have the test. In the past few days I have had increasing difficulty getting fluid into my mouth from the glass, it's the sucking and lip sealing around the edge of the glass that is the problem. On a positive note the speech therapist tells me that everyone thinks I'm doing really well and wonders if it is because I'm keeping so busy. I tend to agree: I'm too busy to dwell on the negative for too long.

The speech therapist mentions that someone else that she has seen with MND has given up. I guess it depends on what you want out of life. There are still a lot of things that I want to do, a lot that I want to achieve. I've waited too long for the opportunities that I have now and I'm not going to give up easily, without a fight.

Tuesday afternoon, after spending the day monitoring at a Sydney hospital, I drive across town to pick up the AFO. The orthotist puts the foot plate into my boot and I put the boot on. Because of the side bar of the AFO it's hard to pull up the zip. Eventually, zip done up, I go for a walk. I feel much more stable. The orthotist suggests that I go for a walk outside to see how I go on uneven ground. Great! I feel almost normal again. Arriving home I try the AFO with my other shoes. The shoes are either too narrow or too small for the foot plate of the AFO and the zips on my boots are too hard to do up without help.

First thing on Wednesday morning I'm off to Christchurch with the AFO safely inside my backpack. Arriving in Christchurch, I check in to the hotel and then with backpack and AFO in hand I head off to find a shoe shop. As I'm walking through the central shopping mall looking for a Hannah's shoe shop I see Ballantynes department store and I think *All the posh old ladies of Christchurch shop here. They're bound to have some suitable shoes*. At the shoe counter I show the sales assistant my note: *I've lost my voice. I need a pair of shoes or ankle boots that I can wear with my foot splint.*

The first couple of shoes are no good. Then we find a pair of plain black leather shoes with a Velcro fastener. The AFO slides in and my foot follows. They are perfect and once on and covered by my trouser leg it looks as though I am wearing a normal pair of shoes - no one would know. I decide to wear the shoes and AFO so I pay for the shoes and off I go with my new found stability, or should I say my old stability back again.

The carbon fiber rod up the side of the leg has a bar at the top which fits around the front of my shin and is held in place by a Velcro fastening strap. As I am walking back to my hotel the carbon fiber bar starts to dig into my shin. I can feel that it will soon rub my shin raw. I pop into *The Body Shop* and buy a foam-padded scrubbing mitt. Back at the hotel I turn the mitt inside out so that the smooth inner surface is on the outside. I slip the mitt on the bar of the AFO. It makes all the difference. Later, back in Sydney, I return to the orthotist who adds some more padding to the fastening strap and with a bit of adjustment it is comfortable. After wearing the AFO for a few days I hardly know it's there.

My busy life continues and I spend a couple of days in Melbourne. Arriving on the second morning at the research building, I find everyone standing in the foyer. Someone tells me that I can't go in because the building has been evacuated. I join the group and wait. As more people arrive I overhear conversations. "The basement has been flooded and the power is off." "The contractors on the building site next door have burst a water main." Some people decide to walk up the stairs to their offices, but there is no way I am going to walk up to the fifth floor with my suitcase, computer bag and backpack, so I wait. Eventually the study coordinator arrives. As well as the power, the computer network is down she can't work in her office. She suggests that we go over to their old office in the hospital and offers to take one of my bags for me. I'm soon settled at a desk with my laptop writing up my reports. By lunchtime, however, when no one had been allowed back in to the building and most staff had been told to go home, I decide to return to Sydney early. I'll be back in Melbourne in a few weeks time and I arrange to finish off the monitoring then.

Kevin is spending Easter in Sydney with me and I'm up early the following morning to collect him from the airport. On Easter Saturday we catch the train from Kogarah in to Circular Quay and go on a two hour scenic harbour cruise. The boat goes out to the Sydney Heads and then up Middle Harbour and under the Spit Bridge to an area of Sydney that I haven't seen before.

On Sunday we go to Circular Quay again to meet my niece Olivia for lunch. There are lots of lovely restaurants outside on the Quay beside the Opera House and I choose one that serves fish, thinking that it will be easy to eat. Kevin and I order Marlin. When the meals arrive the Marlin has been lightly seared on the outside but the middle is raw! I can't eat this. I say to Kevin. He calls the waiter over and we ask if the fish can be cooked. When they bring the fish back it is cooked right through, very tender and I can eat it fairly easily.

Although Olivia has been living in Sydney for less than one year we haven't seen her for a couple of years so there is a bit to catch up on. I keep the conversation going by writing down questions or asking Kevin to explain things. A few days later I have an email from my brother Gavin, Olivia's dad:

> Olivia said that you can hardly talk now. Is it time you came back to live in NZ?

And I reply:

> I really am OK here. My place is easy to manage and close to the airport. I'm usually away for several days each week and I couldn't travel so much if I was in Auckland, it takes too long to get to the airport and I would get too tired. Have a talk to Kevin He has seen how easy everything here is for me.

While he was here Kevin did realise how easy it is for me to manage. I'm sure if I was back in Auckland I would find things much harder to manage and I would get to the stage where it was easier to just give up.

The day that Kevin arrived in Sydney I had a check up appointment with the respiratory physician. "You still look the same, you haven't changed since I first saw you one year ago" he says. "You wondered if you would still be here this Easter, it looks as though you will still be here next Easter." I didn't remind him that one year ago he advised me to give up my job and go back to my family in Auckland.

On Tuesday Kevin returns to Auckland and I go to Brisbane. On arrival in Brisbane I collect my suitcase from the baggage carousel and head out to the taxi queue. I get to the head of the queue and the very overweight Aussie taxi driver puts my bags in the boot. By and large I have found the taxi drivers in Brisbane, Adelaide and Perth to be Australian born native speakers of English, who know where they are going without needing to look up the map and are generally very pleasant people. Whereas in Sydney and Melbourne the taxi drivers are often new immigrants for whom English is not their first language, they often need to look up the map to find the destination and they are often bad tempered.

I settle back in the taxi and start to re-organise the things in my backpack. I put my book and jacket in the bottom of the backpack my drinking glass and coffee cup next and then my glasses on the top. The morning traffic in Brisbane is busy and I can feel that the taxi driver is getting frustrated. He swerves sharply from one lane to the other and back again several times trying to get past slow moving trucks. He waves his hands in the air and swears. By the time we arrive at the hospital all I want to do is to pay the driver and get away from him as fast as I can.

I retrieve my bags and pulling them behind me I walk briskly past the Hospital's main entrance, past the Emergency Department and past the new building site to the Clinical Sciences building. I push the button for the elevator. Nothing lights up to indicate if the elevator is coming. I push the button again, still nothing. Several other people come along. Someone mentions that there is something wrong with the elevator buttons. "It's quicker to walk" she says and heads off up the stairs. There is no way I'm carrying my suitcase, computer bag and backpack up five flights of stairs so I persevere, pushing the button until eventually the elevator comes. Arriving on the fifth floor I struggle to open and get through the smoke stop door with my bags. Finally I greet the two study coordinators and settle down in the conference room to start my work. *Where are my glasses?* They aren't at the top of my backpack! In a panic I unpack the contents of my backpack. As it's dawning on me that I must have left my glasses in the taxi one of the study coordinators comes in. "You look very worried" she says. I've left my glasses in the taxi. "I'll phone the taxi company for you" she offers kindly. "Thanks" I reply. Fortunately the electronic taxi receipt has the identification number of the taxi printed on it.

My glasses are found and we arrange for a taxi to bring them to the hospital. Eventually we get a call to say that the taxi driver is waiting for me at the main entrance of the hospital. I rush to the elevator, wait for what seems like ages for the elevator to arrive and hurry to the main entrance of the hospital.

There are four taxis at the taxi rank and I approach the first one. Suddenly I realise that I don't have a pen and paper. I show the driver my I've lost my voice card and try to explain that I'm looking for the taxi driver who has my glasses. I pull a piece of paper out of my handbag and pointing to his pen say "pen." He hands me his pen and I write: Left glasses in taxi. Taxi driver bringing glasses here.

The driver looks perplexed and shakes his head. I go to the driver's window of the next taxi and repeat my request. Again the driver looks perplexed and I move on to the third taxi. This driver is more patient and helpful. I borrow his pen and write: Taxi driver phoned said he is here with my glasses.

The taxi driver calls up on his radio telephone. "They are going to put out a call to see where the driver is" he says. I thank him for his help and wander off to wait by the front door of the hospital, acutely aware of how this must have looked - a mad woman rushing from one taxi to the next shoving a hand written note through the driver's window! Something makes me go inside to the hospital foyer. There I see a man standing with my glasses case in his hands!

I rush up to him pointing to the glasses and saying "My glasses" "Are you Rebecca?" he asks. "My glasses" I repeat and show him my *I've lost my voice* card. Eventually I manage to convince him that they are my glasses even though my name is not Rebecca. Rebecca is the person who made the phone call for me. What a nightmare.

The rest of the two-day monitoring visit goes smoothly and at 4pm on Wednesday afternoon I go to the taxi rank to get a cab to the airport. The driver recognises me, it's the helpful third driver from yesterday. "Did you get your glasses back?" he asks. "Yes" I reply. At the airport I check in using one of the new quick check-in machines and head to the Qantas Club to wait for my flight back to Sydney.

I'm sitting at one of the long low glass topped benches with my laptop plugged in to the internet answering emails. Three casually dressed guys come and sit opposite me, drinking beer, talking and laughing, I wish they would go away. It's time to take my Riluzole. I look around, but all the seating areas are full and there doesn't appear to be a quiet spot where I can discreetly take my tablet. So I get set up, glass of water, paper serviette, break the tablet in half and pop the first half in my mouth, swig of water and swallow. Down it goes first pop! The second half goes down too without too much coughing and spluttering.

Even though I have effectively lost my voice, I am still leading a full and busy life. I am anxious that people realise that I have lost my voice but I'm not deaf or retarded. A lot of the people I work with have known me well for years and know why I can't talk.

However, there are a few doctors who don't know me well. I'm aware of the impact of first impressions and I'm anxious that they don't get the wrong idea when they meet me.

At one hospital I go with the study coordinator to the cath lab to count the study devices. I know that we might meet the investigator, a doctor whom I don't know well. I write a note If we see him tell him I've lost my voice so he doesn't think I'm mad.

Later in the cath lab the doctor walks in and starts talking to me. I show him my note: If we see him tell him I've lost my voice so he doesn't think I'm mad. "It's OK I know" he says. At another hospital the investigator unexpectedly comes into the room. I don't know him well and I hastily write: I can't speak. "Yes I know" he replies.

On other occasions I know that people have thought that I am mentally retarded. For example one day in March while I am in Perth my mobile phone rings "Hello Barbara, this is Qantas. The departure time of your flight back to Sydney has changed. The new departure time is 11:10am." "OK, can you send me an email" I reply. "The new departure time is 11:10am" the lady repeats. "OK" I say again. The following day my mobile phone rings again. This time it's a man. "I'm just phoning to make sure you know that the departure time of your flight back to Sydney has changed," he says. "Yes I know" I reply. Later a third person from Qantas phones to check that I know the flight time has changed. I am sure they think that I'm mentally retarded or something, but I wonder why they don't just send a text message to my mobile. There must be lots of people out there who have trouble speaking on the phone for one reason or another.

On another occasion I'm at home in Sydney having lunch with friends who are passing through on their way back to England. My mobile rings. It's a man from a company that we work with. He starts asking me about a project that we are working on. I interrupt "Can you send me an email?" I ask. He doesn't understand me and keeps talking. I hand the phone to Loretta and write

Tell him I can't talk. Ask him to send an email. Later I get an email:

> Sorry about persisting with the call, from now on will communicate via email. I did meet you briefly in December and I did know about your voice, again apologies for not opting earlier in the call to use email to communicate.

Early in May I am in Melbourne for several days. I stay at the Hilton hotel for the first two nights.

On my first evening I order a room service dinner by delivering a hand written note to the reception desk. One hour later when the meal has not arrived, I am just leaving the room to go down to reception with a note asking where my dinner is when as I open the door a girl arrives with it. I show her my note and emphasise *One Hour!* She kindly says "No charge for the meal." However, when I check out I notice on my account that I have been charged for the meal after all but I don't say anything, it's just too hard to make a fuss.

On the second night at about 10pm I'm in bed with the light off and just about asleep when there is a knock at the door. I ignore it thinking that it is the room next door. Then after the second knock the door opens and the light is turned on. I leap out of bed to find a foreign looking man in a blue boiler suit coming in to the room. "Did you report a faulty ......" he starts to ask. "NO!" I shout in a loud slurred voice and I slam the door in his face. I get back into bed and go to sleep. Usually hotel staff say who they are when they knock, for example "room service." I don't report the incident to the hotel management because I can't use the phone and I don't want to get dressed and go down to the reception desk. In the morning I'm busy checking out and I don't mention the incident.

For my last night in Melbourne I stay at a cheaper hotel and I do make a fuss. On arrival at the hotel I am faced with a double flight of stairs to the front entrance of the hotel. The taxi driver kindly carries my bags up the stairs for me. When I check in I show the receptionist my *I've lost my voice* card.' The following morning when I check out the same girl is on the reception desk. I write a note asking her to call a taxi for me. I ask her for help to carry my bags down the stairs. "Wait here, the taxi driver will come up" she says. Fifteen minutes later I'm still waiting for the taxi and I write the receptionist a note asking her to check when the taxi was coming. By now I am running late. "Just wait" she says loudly in a tone that makes me think that she thinks I'm deaf. I write *I'm not deaf*. "I know" she says condescendingly. *Or retarded!!* I add. She continues to speak to me as if I am an idiot. I write *I do know, I travel every week for work*. Just then a man smoking a cigarette, starts to walk up the stairs. "Taxi?" I ask. He doesn't understand so I write *Taxi?* He nods. "Help me" I ask pointing to my bags at the top of the stairs. He ignores me and goes back to his taxi which is parked a little further along the road. I hurry down the stairs with my computer bag and then I go back up the stairs to get my suitcase. I really struggle to get my case down the stairs, at the same time being careful not to fall. The receptionist and several Asian tourists in the hotel lobby watch, as does the taxi driver, but no one helps me. I won't be going back there again.

A couple of days later I travel to Auckland to attend the New Zealand Regional Annual Scientific Meeting of the Cardiac Society of Australia and New Zealand held at the Sky City Convention Centre. We are managing the New Zealand sites for a first-in-man clinical trial of a new cardiac device. People who are suitable for enrolment in this trial are hard to find and the trial is enrolling very slowly. In an attempt to identify potentially suitable patients from other parts of the country the device company has decided to publicise the trial by having a booth at the trade exhibition. I send an email offering to assist with the booth:

> I'm willing to take my turn on the booth (I've done this before). Even though I have now effectively lost my voice, a lot of people, including out of town cardiologists, know me and will stop to talk. I can communicate with them by writing and certainly can pass information about the trial on to them.

Madness or not, I am confident that I can attract people to the booth and give them information about the trial. My only concern is that people who don't know me will not know that I can't talk. In advance I email Larry, the representative from the company in the United States who is coming out to represent the company on the booth, just to make sure that he doesn't get the wrong impression when he meets me:

> I think you know that I have now effectively lost my voice, I have motor neurone disease (MND or ALS). Most people know now. I'm well known to a lot of people who will be at the conference, including out of town cardiologists and nurses and they will stop to talk. I can communicate with them by writing and certainly can pass information about the trial on to them.

At the conference I stick a typewritten note to my conference name tag **"Talk to me – I've lost my voice."**

It is really great to catch up with friends and former colleagues, most of whom I have seen periodically throughout the year in the course of my work. They all ask the same question "How are you?" After scribbling my response on note paper several times, I write the following on the cover of my notebook:

> Still in SYD
> Can't talk
> Almost can't swallow
> Otherwise OK
> Working FT + + + !
> Will carry on as long as I can
> Return to AKL when I can't manage

I carry my notebook and pen wherever I go and carry out conversations by writing my questions or responses. I don't feel silly or self conscious - what choice do I have? To hide away in the booth and be invisible? Or to get out there and talk to people?

The three days are very busy. As well as attending the conference on Friday, Saturday and Sunday, Kevin and I go to my sister's housewarming party on Saturday night although we don't stay long. On Sunday night Emma and her family and

Mum come for dinner to celebrate Aaliyah's fourth birthday. Fortunately Kevin does the cooking. He cooks roast pork, and I surprise myself by eating ravenously and reasonably quickly for me.

On Sunday night once everyone has gone home I am exhausted and I'm really pleased that having booked myself on a lunch time flight back to Sydney, I can sleep in on Monday morning.

Arriving in Sydney I collect my suitcase and walk to the taxi rank. Getting into the taxi, I show the Asian driver my *I've lost my voice* card and the card with my address written on it. He indicates to the taxi controller that he has a short fare and proceeds to consult his map. "I live there" I say, unsure of whether or not he can understand me as my voice sounds more like a series of grunts. The traffic is heavy and the taxi driver is getting frustrated and he starts swearing. As we approach the intersection of West Botany Road and President Avenue he asks if he should turn right by making grunting noises and pointing right. I indicate that we should turn right. It's after 3pm and the right hand turn from President Avenue into the Princes Highway is controlled by tidal flow lights. In the evening rush hour only the right lane of the three lanes can turn right whereas at other times the middle lane can also make a right hand turn. The taxi driver remains in the middle lane. At this time of the day the middle lane must turn left. I start to indicate that he needs to be in the right lane and he hands me some paper to write on. I write *only R lane turn right*. He starts to make more grunting noises and remains in the middle lane. After two changes of lights we turn right and first left into Kensington street. Again the driver grunts and points left to ask if we should turn left. We get to a roundabout in the road and he grunts "errr errr?" Asking if we go straight ahead. When we get to Belgrave Street I point right and say "right here." Again he grunts "errrr errrr." When we stop outside my building he grunts "errrr errrr." I pay my fare, feeling rather insulted that he seems to be making fun of the way I talk. The only redeeming thing is that he carries my bags across the road for me. Am I just unlucky? Or does everyone have trouble with taxi drivers? I feel as though I should be writing a book called *My experiences with taxi drivers in Australia and New Zealand.*

The next morning I'm up early to go to Melbourne again for a training session for a new study. Two American women are in Melbourne to conduct the training and I join them for lunch. I usually avoid eating with clients because I'm so slow and it's just too hard but one of these ladies has an aunt who, following surgery, has difficulty speaking and swallowing and she understands my situation. Later in the evening we join a colleague from Melbourne for dinner. We have a truly lovely evening and I'm glad that I had the courage to join them. Later I send them an email:

> It was great to get to meet you both at last, and I enjoyed the dinner on Wednesday night very much, I haven't laughed so much for a long time!
>
> Thanks for being patient with me.

And the reply from the Director of Clinical Programs

> It was wonderful meeting you as well last week. I think that you will be able to provide the kind of support and guidance that the young study coordinator needs as she continues to grow. I also appreciate your guidance as I do strive to learn from other people's clinical trial experience, and you have quite a lot!

And from her boss: Ditto to all! Cheers!

11

Cough as a presenting symptom of MND

The single most distressing and persistent symptom of MND that I have suffered is a cough. I feel that the first episodes of coughing signified the beginning of my symptoms of MND.

Back in 2001 I had two episodes of coughing. The first was in May while I was at a meeting in Durham, North Carolina, and the second episode began in Stockholm and I continued to cough intermittently throughout a three week Scandinavian trip, which incidentally spanned the 9/11 events in the USA and the subsequent tightening of airline security. A few years earlier my Auckland GP told me that the cough waking me in the night was bronchospasm, or asthma, and prescribed a ventolin inhaler. The cough that I had in 2001 occurred only in the day and I assumed it was bronchospasm, the same cough, triggered in North Carolina by the spring pollen on the pine trees that surrounded the hotel where I was staying. Similarly, I assumed that the cough that plagued me in Sweden was triggered by cigarette smoke. People in Stockholm were smoking everywhere. There was no such thing as a smoke-free section in a restaurant. The cough was not relieved by use of my ventolin inhaler.

Over the next few years I had increasing episodes of coughing.

The cough was always dry and unproductive. There was a tickle in my throat. Sometimes I felt as though there was a plug of mucus in my throat and if I could only cough it out I would stop coughing. I particularly remember when I moved to Sydney in June 2003 standing in line at the immigration counter at Sydney airport and trying hard not to cough. At the time the world was in fear of the outbreak of SARS in Asia. Completing my SARS questionnaire to be presented to the immigration officer, knowing that I did not have SARS, I had checked NO to the question 'Do you have a cough?'

The cough was never relieved by using my ventolin inhaler. However, it was eased by sucking throat lozenges, particularly 'Throaties.' I never went anywhere without some 'Throaties' and at work I got into the habit of popping one into my mouth before going into a meeting.

As time went on the episodes of coughing became more frequent and by mid 2004 I would sometimes cough for several hours at a time. My Auckland GP wanted to refer me to a respiratory physician, but I was never in Auckland for long enough. A medical colleague kept saying "You need steroids."

Eventually, as mentioned earlier, I saw a Sydney GP who referred me to an ENT surgeon who quickly dismissed the cough and focused on my husky voice. When I did eventually have a formal respiratory assessment in Sydney in 2005 as described earlier I was coughing so much that I had difficulty doing the breathing tests and the physician said that I had asthma. I started to use the steroid and bronchial dilator inhalers religiously, strictly as prescribed in an attempt to rid myself of the cough.

"Using the inhaler triggers my cough" I said to the respiratory physician the next time I saw him. "You need to use a spacer" he replied. "A spacer is a plastic chamber between the inhaler and your mouth. This allows you to press the inhaler and then take a breath when you are ready," he said. But even using the spacer, as soon as the inhaled air hit the back of my throat I coughed, effectively coughing out some of the medication. So the cough continued. It did not get better; if anything it got worse.

Sometimes I would be free of the cough for days on end. Other times I would cough for days on end. Talking makes me cough. I particularly remember that the week in April 2005 that I spent in Melbourne training Judy, a new CRA from Japan, I was plagued by coughing. I felt particularly bad because there was so much that I could teach Judy. But I could not speak without coughing.

A couple of months later, arriving back in Sydney one evening I started coughing. Well, really, the cough started during the flight from Christchurch. Every time I breathed out I coughed and this went on for several hours. It got worse and I was beginning to get worried. I had rapid shallow breathing. And every time I breathed out there was an awful grunting noise. I thought about going to the emergency department of the St George Hospital which is at the end of the street that I live in. But in the end I decided just to go to bed and see what would happen. Once in bed I relaxed and the coughing stopped.

This episode has given me a fright though. I feel so insecure because I don't seem to be able to control the cough with medication. The cough lozenges do ease it but only temporarily. So I deicide to stop using the asthma inhalers because they haven't been working anyway.

A week or so later I get an email from Margie, the nurse coordinator at the motor neurone disease clinic.

> Have there been any concerning issues? Anything I can help with? Swallowing? Speech? Weakness?

I reply:

> I am managing very well. My speech is variable, swallowing variable too but I am able to swallow my tablets (with care) and can still manage regular fluids. I have still been very troubled by a dry cough that the respiratory physician thought was asthma but the inhaled steroid and bronchodilator has not helped. I have used the inhalers strictly as instructed since they were prescribed but if anything the cough was worse - so I have not taken them for a week and so far the cough has been much better. I think my left foot is weaker like my left hand but I can still walk briskly past everyone in the airport terminals!

Margie replies:

> If you want another ENT opinion, there is an ENT specialist here at POWH. He recently saw one of our patients who also has Bulbar MND with some of the same symptoms (actually a little

> worse) and he appears to be good. We haven't had too much to do with him, but if you wanted to we could try and get you in to see him. (This other patient will be having botox to hopefully alleviate her symptoms/ laryngospasm). I'll let you think about it, and you can let me know.

On reading Margie's reply suddenly the penny drops. *"That's what is causing the cough, I'm sure of it."* I reply indicating that I would like to see this ENT surgeon.

I do a quick internet search for laryngospasm and motor neurone disease. Pretty soon I find an 87 page document entitled *Ethics, Communication and Decision Making, Appendix C.* There is no indication of the origin of the document and it seems to be a collection of papers on the findings of working groups. I quickly find what I am looking for under the heading 'Symptoms indirectly caused by ALS':

Laryngospasm (a sudden reflectory closure of the vocal cords) can cause panic because of the sensation of choking. Several types of stimuli (e.g. emotions, strong flavors or smells, cold air, fluid aspiration, sinus drainage or gastroesophageal reflux) may provoke this symptom, which usually resolves spontaneously within a few seconds. Repeated swallowing while breathing through the nose can accelerate resolution. Patients also benefit from reassurance and education about this distressing symptom. H1 H2 blocking agents (antihistamines or antacids) also may be helpful in selected patients.[1]

On my written list of symptoms that was ignored by the ENT surgeon who I saw in August 2004 I wrote: Intermittent cough during the day, worse as the day progresses. Triggers: cigarette smoke, perfumes, pollens, laughing and stressful situations, diagnosed as bronchospasm.

I am surprised that none of the doctors that I have seen since my diagnosis has picked this up. I have mentioned my cough several times. "It could be caused by aspiration of food or fluid" was one response. There has never been any intensive questioning on the exact nature of the cough, what triggers it and what relieves it.

When I mentioned to close medical colleagues that my asthma inhalers didn't relieve the cough none of them suggested that the cough could be caused by laryngospasm. But then why would they? They are not neurologists. They have no specialist knowledge of MND.

The cough eventually settles and I don't pursue Margie's suggestion to see the specialist at POWH. At the same time, however, my speech deteriorates to the stage where I can only say a few words. I am so pleased to no longer be troubled by the cough, but I feel that the cough has robbed me of many months of good verbal communication had I not been coughing.

Suddenly, out of the blue, in June 2006 a week after the PEG insertion I start coughing again. It's the same cough, starting as a tickle in the throat. Every time I exhale I cough or grunt. Again 'Throaties' help. By now I have a soft supportive neck collar and wearing the collar also helps. I'm convinced that the cough is part of the symptoms of MND. I search the internet for 'Cough as a presenting symptom in MND' and 'Cough as a presenting symptom in ALS'. *Why haven't I done this earlier?* I wonder.

Almost straight off I find a paper: *Vocal cord dysfunction: Paradoxical vocal cord motion - A thorough review.* It's a summary of a Grand Round presentation by Todd M Wiess, a senior medical student. Causes of paradoxical vocal cord motion (PVDM) include cortical injury involving either upper or lower motor neurons. Symptoms include cough, inspiratory/expiratory wheeze, dyspnoea with or without exercise, stridor, hoarseness and reflux, all of which I've had at some time or other. In a study of people with PVDM, cough was found to be the most common feature.[2]

The paper goes on to describe adduction or "chinking" of the vocal cord during inspiration or early expiration.[2] I can breathe in all right, it's when I start to breathe out that something in my throat catches and I cough and sometimes I make a grunting sound. This occurs with every breath and can sometimes go on for several hours.

There are many causes of PVDM and it is more common in young and middle aged women. Maybe the ENT surgeon that I saw was right when he said to me "Your vocal cords are not moving properly when you talk." However, what he didn't do was to consider the cause of the PVDM. PVDM can be caused by a range of diseases including MND/ALS. The paper also mentions that PVDM is often mis-diagnosed as asthma.[2]

Triggers for PVDM include smoke, perfume and emotional stress.[2] When the cough first started I was sharing my office with another study coordinator. I noticed that every morning when she came in I could smell her perfume and I would start coughing. Also I would start coughing in smoky rooms and stressful situations triggered the cough.

At about the same time as the cough started I had several tearful episodes that at the time I attributed to stressful situations. However, in retrospect it was unusual for me to cry in these situations and I suspect that the tears were related to the onset of bulbar symptoms of MND.

For me the two most distressing symptoms of MND have been the incessant and distressing coughing and the unpredictable and uncontrollable episodes of crying. Both have been largely glossed over or mis-interpreted.

I also suspect that the episodes of uncontrollable excessive yawning that I first experienced in 2003 are another early symptom of MND. These attacks of yawning were a source of acute embarrassment to me as they often occurred during meetings. As a new staff member at the Sydney pharmaceutical company I was keen to learn and participate in the meetings. I was certainly not bored or tired.

The attacks of yawning continue to occur and it is only recently that I have linked them to MND. One evening while watching a medical drama on television it is mentioned that the patient's yawning has a neurological cause. *Maybe that's why I yawn so much* I think. Searching the internet for 'yawning and MND'

I find several references to yawning and MND. People with bulbar onset MND commonly have "attacks of uncontrollable yawning, sometimes when they are not even tired."[3]

1 *Communication and Decision Making. Appendix C.* http://www. promotingexcellence.org/files/public/als_appendix_c.pdf accessed 7th Apr 2007.

2 Todd M Weiss (2001) *Vocal Cord Dysfunction: Paradoxical Vocal Cord Motion - a thorough review.* Source: Grand Rounds Presentation, UTMB, Department of Otolaryngology. Grand Rounds Index: UTMB Otolaryngology index. http://www.utmb.edu/otoref/grnds/Vocal-Cord-2001-07/VCD-2.htm accessed 7 Apr 2007.

3 Wicks, Paul. *Excessive yawning is common in the bulbar-onset form of ALS.* Acta Psychiatr Scand , 0705220158 (Tue May 22 00:00:00 UTC 2007) DOI:(10.1111/j.1600-0447.2007.01025) http://www.blackwell-synergy.com/doi/abs/10.1111/j.1600-0447.2007.01025.x?journalCode=acp accessed 30 June 2007.

12

PEG'd - June 2006

Up till now apart from medication I've managed to be able to live normally without medical intervention or devices. I know that the medical literature says that Percutaneous Endoscopic Gastrostomy (PEG) Non Invasive Positive Pressure Ventilation (NIPPV) both prolong survival, but it's hard to accept. In a way I feel that it's like the beginning of the end.

After my MND clinic appointment on 21st March the appointments with the orthotist for the AFO and the speech therapist for the modified barium swallow follow fairly quickly and I am able to see the respiratory specialist before Easter. Then things get in the way. I have monitoring visits to Christchurch, Melbourne and Brisbane, and the Easter and Anzac Day holidays and school holidays disrupt schedules.

After the modified barium swallow I elect to have follow up and ongoing management locally at Calvary and St George Hospitals rather than at the Prince of Wales Hospital which is a 20-30 minute drive away. In addition, parking at the Prince of Wales Hospital costs me $15 each time, whereas parking is free at Calvary and I can walk to St George.

My appointment with the palliative care doctor is initially scheduled for Monday April 24th which is ideal because I have two weeks at home before my next round of out of town travel. However, on the day of the appointment I get an email postponing the appointment:

> She wondered if she could re book you for next Monday...at 2:30 or if the morning is better she can make a time to suit you.

The following Monday I arrive at Calvary hospital at 2:25 and while I'm busy writing a note for the receptionist asking where the clinic is the palliative care doctor comes along. "Hello Barbara, I was just leaving." This surprises me because my appointment is for 2:30 and I'm not late. Anyway we walk back to the clinic and the consultation goes ahead.

We discuss my need for a PEG and she agrees that I do need one. I'm hoping that I can have the PEG insertion this week because I'm going to Melbourne on Sunday and will be away for the next two weeks I write. "There isn't time" she replies. "You will need to stay in hospital overnight and you really need to have a week at home afterwards. It can be quite painful and there is a risk of infection."

I tell her that I'll be back in Sydney on May 22nd and we agree that that I should have the PEG insertion that week. She will send a referral letter to the gastroenterologist at St George Hospital. I have several questions regarding PEG insertion and management and she says that she will ask Margie to talk to me.

I'm disappointed that I have to wait another two weeks. I've really been struggling with my tablets for about six months. Before Christmas I thought, *well it's only a couple of months before my next MND clinic appointment. I'll need a PEG by then.* Time has gone on and it looks like I won't get the PEG until the end of May!

The next day is Tuesday May 2 and my sleep test is scheduled for 7pm in the evening. Originally the sleep test was booked for May 22nd but I had asked for an earlier appointment if a slot comes up because of a cancellation, and I am lucky.

Knowing that I need to be at the Prince of Wales Hospital by 7 pm, I take my Riluzole half an hour early at 4:30 and start eating my dinner one hour later at 5:30. I need to leave home at 6:15. I'm eating so slowly these days that by 6:15 I'm only half way through my meal. I make a sandwich of the rest of the meal and take it with me.

Arriving at the sleep clinic at 7pm, I'm shown to a room. I need to finish my dinner I write. I sit down by the bed and start eating my sandwich. The technician comes back into the room. "I've put you in the wrong room" she says, so I pack up my things and shift to another room. It takes me a couple of trips to move everything. It takes me about 30 minutes to finish eating, and I'm hurrying because I know that they are waiting to put the electrodes on and this process takes quite a while.

Eventually I'm finished and I go into another room for the electrodes to be put on. First she takes my blood pressure. "Your blood pressure is up a bit" she says. I've been rushing to get here. I write in reply. An understatement really. It's been quite stressful getting my work finished, preparing and eating dinner, driving to the hospital, then eating my sandwich and taking my evening tablets with spoonfuls of trifle that I brought with me in a jar!

All wired up, I return to my room, get into bed and read my book. Having taken my Amitriptyline with its sedative effect, I start to feel sleepy. By about 10pm I decide to try and go to sleep. There are electrodes behind each ear so no matter which side I lie on they dig in, and the tubing from the nasal prongs is tucked behind my ears adding to the discomfort. No matter which side I lie on I just can't get comfortable and I toss and turn for what seems like hours before finally falling asleep.

I wake once in the night and again toss and turn for about one hour before falling asleep again. At about 4am another patient rings his buzzer and this wakes me again. I can't go back to sleep. I have asked to be woken at 5am so that I can take my Riluzole and then I need to go home as I have a teleconference at 7am.

In the morning I think *this sleep test is no better than the one I had last year.* Maybe I went to sleep a bit quicker, but well over the 40 minutes (more like two hours) which is the maximum time on the morning questionnaire. The evening questionnaire includes a somnolence assessment, I score one (0 being the best). As I am filling it in I think *I know several people who would easily get a much higher score than me.*

I complete the morning questionnaire. In response to the question 'How well did you sleep?' I check the option 'Much worse than usual.' The reason for having a sleep test is to diagnose breathing problems that occur during sleep. If normal sleeping patterns are disrupted breathing problems such as apnoea may not occur. I really can't understand why more importance is not placed on ensuring maximum comfort during the sleep test. I have been so uncomfortable and unable to sleep well at both sleep tests that I am really very tempted to decline if I need to have another one.

I spend the rest of the week in Sydney working at home and on Thursday I have a monitoring visit at a local Sydney Hospital. By Saturday morning I have caught up on my sleep, I'm up to date with my work, and preparing for the next two weeks. I am off to Melbourne on Sunday afternoon, back to Sydney on Wednesday evening, Auckland Friday morning, back to Sydney Monday afternoon and back again to Melbourne on Tuesday for the rest of the week.

During the week I get an email from Margie:

> I was wondering when you would be free for me to pop over and go through some PEG questions that you may have? I am going to work for half a day this Saturday (6th May), so if you are in Sydney I can pop in, otherwise give me some dates that you are around and I'll work something out.

As it happens, Margie is running behind in her home visits on Saturday and doesn't come and see me so I email her an update and attach my list of questions:

> Hi Margie, I've attached a list of my questions regarding PEG insertion and management.
>
> I really think that I have needed it for some time, possibly as early as February. I had been hoping to get it done during these past 2 weeks while I have been in Sydney but that wasn't possible.
>
> I have a very busy 2 weeks in Melbourne with meetings, and dinners with 2 different groups of visiting Americans, from

> medical device companies – I'm not sure if I'll make it to the dinners. In the middle of it I have a cardiology conference in Auckland next weekend where I will be manning a publicity booth with an American man from the device company in USA. Most people who will be at the conference have known me for years. The Americans have been very understanding and helpful. They have all got to know me via email communication so that when we meet it's not so difficult.
>
> I would like PEG insertion to be early in the week of May 22. I can arrange to be in Sydney for a week. They have contacted the gastroenterologist at St George (public) but I haven't been sent an appointment or anything yet.
>
> They were also organising for me to see the rehab man at Calvary but I haven't received an appointment for that yet. The lady at reception has my email address and she knows that I'm away for the next 2 weeks.
>
> The sleep test was on Tues May 2 and I have a follow up appointment on May 23.
>
> I'll be going away again for work probably the last week of May starting May 29 and will probably be away for a few days most weeks in June.

A few days later I get an email advising me that I am unable to be fitted in at St George hospital for the PEG insertion until August. It is suggested that I consider having it done at Prince of Wales Hospital.

In my response I mention that I originally elected to have the PEG at St George because it is so close and I can walk there and back, whereas at Prince of Wales Hospital I will need to get a taxi there and back again as I will have no one here at home with me, and I won't be able to drive immediately after the PEG insertion. The procedure at Prince of Wales Hospital involves an outpatient's appointment, followed a week or two later by the PEG insertion, done as a day procedure, and then another follow up appointment. I can see this dragging out till July or August. For ongoing support St George is also much more convenient. I really don't want to have to keep going backwards and forwards to Prince of Wales Hospital. I'm just too busy.

I am beginning to feel as though I am getting the run around. I think that I have needed a PEG since the beginning of 2006. Initially I was waiting till I had my MND clinic appointment in March and the subsequent modified Barium swallow which was on 3 April. Now it looks as though I might not get it until August! It's almost as though no one is taking me seriously, that if I'm still working full time and travelling around the country every week I must be OK.

My main problems are with taking tablets and drinking. With drinking it's the lip seal. About half of what I'm drinking comes out down the front of my shirt or into a serviette or towel, which isn't terribly nice when I'm with other people. As mentioned earlier I am having great difficulty swallowing tablets and sometimes I vomit. I can usually manage to eat enough, although by meal times I am feeling hungry and I never used to feel hungry, and I know that I'm not eating the right food.

When I mention to a former colleague, now friend, that I need a PEG and BiPAP he says "You remain a battling inspiration." At about the same time another friend asks "Don't you want to stop work, spend some time at home, or travel while you still can?" But really what option do I have? If I stopped work what would I do? All my friends are working and I would just sit at home feeling miserable and dwelling on all the negative things. I think that there is a limit to where and for how long I could travel. It would mean giving up my job and once I had exhausted my ready cash where would I be? No job, short of money and again the prospect of sitting at home feeling miserable. Besides I love my job and if I quit now I know that I would regret it. I'm still getting messages of support when I introduce myself by email to companies we are starting to work with. Just today this email arrived:

> Dear Barbara,
> It is very nice to meet you and I look forward to working with you on this project. I am sorry to hear about ALS, but it sounds

> like you are taking things in stride. I'm sure email would end up being the preferred communication method anyway, due to the time differences, etc..........

Just when I am beginning to despair of ever getting the PEG inserted, I have another email from Margie saying that a different gastroenterologist at St George Hospital might be able to fit me in to his list for PEG insertion. A few days later I'm given a date: June 7. This suits my work plans. On Tuesday June 6 I'm at home working, waiting to be told when to go in to the hospital. At 11am I get a text message from Margie saying that there aren't any beds available and she will get back to me later in the day. It's winter in Sydney and I'm very aware of the 'winter bed state' in public hospitals in New Zealand-Australian public hospitals aren't any different. Each winter the medical beds fill up with people suffering winter illnesses. This often has a flow-on effect to the surgical and other wards in the hospitals, and hospitals are frequently closed for admissions, even turning away ambulances with acutely ill patients.

Then at 4:30pm I get a phone call from Margie. "There is a bed available for you in Ward 3 North" and she tells me to go straight there. I'm all packed ready and waiting so I quickly have my 5pm Riluzole tablet, email my boss to say I have a bed and I walk up the road to the main entrance of the hospital.

Knowing what information in the way of past history, current medication etc. is required I've taken several typed sheets of information with me. One for the admitting doctor, one for the anaesthetist and one for the dietician. The admitting doctor is a young intern and he is pleased to have the information. He asks me why I am taking the tablets. This is quite reasonable as he probably has not encountered a patient with MND before. I don't see any other doctors that evening and I go to sleep wondering what the morning will bring.

Well, actually, I don't sleep. This is the first time in my life that I have been in hospital as a patient overnight. (I don't count the two sleep tests as they are day case visits that just happen to be at night!) Having spent most of my working life in hospitals, though, I am well aware that the activity in the ward continues during the night. This night is no exception. Infusion pumps are constantly alarming and patients ring their buzzers all night. I have never known patients to buzz for the nurse so much before! Then there is a confused elderly man in the room across the corridor who keeps swearing all night and calling for the nurse. On top of all of this the mattress on my bed feels like it is full of concrete. Knowing that the Amitriptyline I have taken has a sedative effect, I don't ask for a sleeping pill. Acutely aware of my compromised overnight respiratory status, I don't want to further depress my breathing.

In the morning the registrar arrives with the consent form for me to sign. I understand his explanations of the procedure and the associated risks and he asks if I have any questions. I write PEG exit point to avoid waistband area. "Show this note to the doctor when you see him outside the endoscopy theatre" he replies. What sort of an anaesthetic will I have? I ask. "It's a heavy sedation and you won't remember what happened" he says. I haven't been seen by the anaesthetist yet and I'm assured that I will also see him outside the endoscopy theatre. I sign the consent form and wait to be wheeled down to the theatre.

In the waiting area the gastroenterologist comes and checks my abdomen and I show him my note PEG exit point to avoid waistband area. He says something about the exit point being dependant on the anatomy, so I just hope for the best. Then the anaesthetist comes along. I show her my note I'm waiting for overnight BiPAP to start. Lung function deteriorating. Supposed to have anaesthetic review before PEG. My more detailed handwritten note is still in the ward because I am expecting the anaesthetist to have received a copy of my latest respiratory tests. She glances at my medical notes and looks perplexed. In a panic I indicate that I want pen and paper to write something. She goes away and comes back with a black felt pen and a piece of paper. I write:

Registrar has fax of respt status
- tidal vol
- overnight O2 Sats
apnoea

This is sufficient to alert her to my compromised respiratory function and she says "We'll put a tube down." That's what I wanted. My two concerns about this procedure are firstly that the PEG tube will be inserted at waistband level and will constantly cause me discomfort and secondly that under heavy sedation I will stop breathing and no one will notice. With a tube down, I'll be ventilated so that I don't stop breathing and my airway will be protected from aspirating any saliva or gastric fluid.

Over the past year or so in the course of my work I have watched several cardiac procedures where devices are inserted using TOE (trans-oesophageal echo) guidance. PEG tubes are inserted using gastroscopic guidance. In both cases a black hose about finger thickness is inserted via the mouth into the oesophagus (TOE) or the stomach (gastroscopy). The cardiac procedures are done using a general anaesthetic or sedation and local, depending on the condition of the patient. I formed the opinion then that I would not like to have this done under local.

I'm wheeled into the endoscopy theatre, a man says "Hello I'm another anaesthetist. I'm just going to pop this (IV cannula) into your arm." I indicate that I want it in the other arm, a little prick and it's in and hooked up to a bag of IV fluid. "I'm just giving you a little sedation" he says and the next thing I know I'm lying on my right side on my bed in the recovery room with an oxygen mask over my nose and mouth and a very sore area on the left side of my abdomen. "We put some local anaesthetic in" someone says, but it must be wearing off.

The afternoon and evening pass in a blur of medication, water infusion running in to the PEG tube, and other patients coming and going. Margie pops in to visit me; she thinks the PEG is sited in a good location. The dietician and nutritional support nurse pop in and say that they will be back tomorrow. I stay awake until I have been given my 10pm antibiotic. By now the IV infusion has stopped and the 10mls of antibiotic is injected directly in to the IV cannula. The nurse pushes it in so quickly that it stings. All the other nurses have given the antibiotic very slowly over about five minutes. In my day all intravenous antibiotic injections were given in 100mls of fluid in a burette chamber and dripped through slowly. We weren't allowed to give antibiotics directly into the vein as a bolus injection.

Despite the fact that the elderly lady in the next bed is having a bowel prep for a colonoscopy the next day and is up all night with diarrhoea and vomiting, I sleep fairly well.

The morning comes and we are woken early. Both mornings the surgical doctors have arrived on the ward at about 7am to see their patients. Coming from a medical/cardiology background where ward rounds don't get underway until 8 or 8:30, I'm impressed. My tummy hurts and its very hard to move around the bed. I cough and it hurts. I remember from my student nurse days that you are supposed to hold your wound when you cough, but this doesn't help much.

I'm getting used to the routine for giving medication via the tube and fairly soon I'm doing it myself and correcting some of the nurses when they start to do something the wrong way. The dietician spends quite a while working out a nutritional plan for me. This includes Jevity Hi-cal, a high fibre/high calorie feed, nutritional supplements and gives scope for me to eat regular food as well.

Someone mentions to me that I'm lucky to have had the PEG done because there are quite a few people waiting to have it done. Yes, I probably am lucky to have had it done. To put this into perspective, though, the PEG will improve my quality of life, improve my nutritional status, possibly slow the rate of muscle loss and hopefully allow me to live independently and continue working for some time longer. Is it too much to ask when my remaining life span may be counted in months or at best maybe a couple of years?

By the time the nutritional support nurse comes back I have just finished giving myself a tin of Jevity Hi-cal and she can see that I am managing well. While I'm waiting for my final antibiotic injection I overhear the daughter of a lady who has just been admitted saying "My mother is non-verbal. She will indicate yes and no but she is definitely non-verbal." *That's a new one* I think, and not a term that I would like to use to describe myself. As soon as I have had my last IV antibiotic, I'm free to go home. Pulling my suitcase behind me I walk around the corner and I'm home.

By lunchtime on Friday I'm sitting at my computer nibbling on a chicken and avocado sandwich and thinking that my stomach isn't used to having so much liquid in it. It's all a bit weird. This whole thing is going to take a bit of getting used to.

What to do with what seems like yards of tubing to hide under my clothing? Initially I strap the tube to my chest with a crepe bandage. A little later while I am at the local shopping mall I spot a rack of lycra stretch 'control' knickers on special at three for $10. Thinking *that'll do* I test the stretch of the lycra and it's OK, not too tight. There is no way it would control rolls of abdominal fat but it's perfect for my intended use. I buy three and at home I cut off the elastic waist band and the leg portions. I'm left with a tube of lycra, just the right size to fit snugly around my lower chest. By placing the PEG tube on the lycra and then folding the lycra over the tube, once from below and then from above the tube sits snugly, just below my bra. It's very comfortable and pretty much invisible under my clothing.

What to do with the tube in the shower? I string it up on a cord around my neck, and that actually works well. I need to turn the tube 360° every day, firstly so that a tract forms (just like when you have your ears pierced) and then to keep the hole there - OUCH! It's really not so bad if I do it in the shower when I'm warm.

I've also been to the dietary department at St George Hospital and bought $69 worth of cans of Jevity Hi-cal. Each 237ml can is supposed to be the same as a meat and veges dinner. The dietician wants me to have two a day so I'll need to take them with me when I travel. She wants me to have two little bottles of Yakult a day, something I would never drink! She also wants me to either eat fish twice a week or have fish oil via the tube. Apparently Omega 3 fatty acids have been found to help in preventing muscle breakdown in MND. I'm sure if I stick to the diet, I'll be getting better nutrition than I've had for ages, but the thought of some of this stuff going into my stomach makes me screw up my nose.

For several days I'm quite tender just above the insertion site. It hurts to bend over. You don't realise how many times you stoop down to pick something up until there is a problem doing it. I've had dreadful cramp-like pains two nights in a row. It's like my stomach is trying to digest or expel the foreign object. There is a plastic bolster in my stomach to stop the tube falling out. But the tube is traction removable, which means that it can be pulled out – OUCH! I swab the insertion site with povidone-iodine, firstly to prevent infection while the wound is healing and then, because it's a direct tract into my stomach, to keep the site reasonably free from the usual bacteria that are on the skin. Then I put a dressing of non-stick pads between the skin and the flange of the tube, firstly to prevent pressure areas and secondly to soak up the small amount of leakage of stomach contents. The non-stick dressing pads come in a box of assorted sizes so I need to cut them to size.

Whilst I'm back working as soon as I'm out of hospital I have been advised not to travel for one week. And in retrospect it is sound advice. We are very busy at work and I really need to be away every week to keep up with things and to meet deadlines. Some time ago I booked a return flight to Auckland using my frequent flyer points to attend the memorial service for Barbara's mother. As it happens I need to be in Auckland for two days and decide to combine the trips. I purchase a return trip to Auckland and try to change my frequent flyer ticket by pushing it forward to the Australian Labour weekend. The Qantas internet reservation system won't let me make the change. There is an email address for Qantas sales at the bottom of the page so I send an email:

> I am contacting you by email because I have lost my voice and I am not able to speak on the phone. This is a permanent loss caused by a medical condition.

> I wish to change the booking (Booking reference 2IAOVR) below made with my frequent flyer points, as in the interim I have to be in Auckland for business and have subsequently purchased a ticket (Booking reference Z4LRH7).

Qantas sales replies:

> Thank you for your Email.
> Fare quotes, reservations, booking changes and cancellations cannot be answered via email.
>
> Please contact your local Qantas office for further assistance with your enquiry. Mrs Williams, am sorry to hear that you have lost your voice, you will need to ask someone to contact them on your behalf.

And I reply:

> Thank you, however I live alone, with no one who can make phone calls for me. There must be others in my situation, maybe they are deaf, who are unable to speak but otherwise lead a very full, busy life and travel frequently. Perhaps Qantas could consider adjusting the booking system to accommodate us?
>
> I do ALL my very frequent travel reservations via the internet.
>
> Will I be able to make this change at the service desk in the International Qantas Club in terminal 1 at Sydney airport when I am on my way to Auckland on Wednesday morning?

Sometime later my mobile phone rings "Hello, this is Qantas, can I speak to Barbara?" I say "Me." The lady repeats "Can I speak to Barbara?" "Me" I repeat, and the lady hangs up. In a few minutes my mobile rings again "Hello, this is Qantas, can I speak to Barbara?" "Me" I say, feeling very frustrated.

I email Qantas sales again

> Someone from Qantas has just phoned me on my mobile phone.
>
> As below I HAVE LOST MY VOICE. PLEASE CONTACT ME BY EMAIL OR TEXT ON MOBILE.

Then in quick succession I receive two emails - e-tickets for booking reference 2IAOVR and the flight that I'm trying to change booking reference Z4LRH7.

Shortly after this I receive another email:

> I believe that they were contacting you in relation to the above bookings which have been duplicated.
>
> Which booking do you wish to be cancelled?

I reply by repeating which flights I want to cancel. Just as I'm thinking that there has to be a better way, I can't be the only Qantas customer in this situation, I receive another email:

> I have contacted our Telephone Sales staff who have changed the above booking to the flights you have requested.
>
> This is able to be done without any charge.
>
> A copy of your new itinerary has been sent via separate Email.
>
> Kind Regards,
> Qantas Network Operations.

Thanks Qantas!! Why wasn't it this easy in the beginning? At times I feel so helpless. Here I am, a busy and competent professional person just trying to get on with life as best as I can while I am able to. There must be so many other people, with various problems, out there trying to do the same.

A few days later I'm on my way to Auckland. In my suitcase I have packed eight tins of Jevity, a small plastic jug, my pill crusher, a small plastic cup for dissolving my medication, a small cocktail fork for mixing the medication and 50ml and 10ml syringes. I've also made copies of my hospital discharge letter, nutritional plan and the dietary prescription for Jevity, thinking that these should be sufficient evidence of the contents of the tins. I don't declare anything on my New Zealand arrivals card. Why should I? I don't have any banned products.

On arrival in Auckland I collect my suitcase and proceed to the agricultural x-ray machine As my suitcase is going through the x-ray machine one of the inspectors asks "What are the tins in your suitcase?" I'm standing beside the x-ray machine and all my bags are disappearing into the machine. I can't speak. I point to the x-ray machine frantically waving my hand to indicate that I want one of the bags inside the machine. By now the man is opening my suitcase. The cans are at the bottom of my case but I know exactly where they are and I rip open the plastic bag and pull out a can. I'm still frantically indicating that I want the other bags which by now are coming out of the x-ray machine.

I open the side pocket of my computer bag pulling out my documentation and thrust it at the man. By now I'm crying out of sheer frustration!!! Then I grab my handbag and pull out my *I've lost my voice* card thrusting it at the man pointing frantically to the words. The man reads the ingredients on the can and then says "They are OK". By now I'm angry, still crying and I write *I know OK*. The other man at the x-ray machine asks "What is it?" "Something from the hospital" the first man replies.

I just don't need this sort of hassle every time I enter New Zealand and I decide to make a new note to take with me when I travel.

I have motor neurone disease

I have lost my voice

I can't swallow and I have a feeding tube into my stomach

The cans are prescribed nutritional formula to take via the stomach tube

The formula is scientifically prepared by Abbott Laboratories (offices in Australia and New Zealand)

On the plane from Sydney to Auckland four young deaf British back packers are sitting in front of me. Throughout the flight they keep up an animated conversation with each other, two leaning over from the row in front to sign and speak silently to the other two. I feel tired just watching them but at the same time I think they look just like any other group of young backpackers away from home on their OE and having a great time. Their deafness is no handicap to them. And I don't consider my inability to speak to be a handicap. Frustrating yes, but I'm certainly not going to let it stop me doing things.

A week later I have a day trip to Melbourne. In my backpack I have one tin of Jevity, a small plastic jug, my pill crusher, a small plastic cup for dissolving my medication, a small cocktail fork for mixing the medication and a 50ml syringe. I have no trouble passing through the security x-ray screening at the Sydney domestic terminal. However, in the afternoon on my way back to Sydney, passing through the security x-ray screening at the Melbourne domestic terminal, as my backpack comes out of the x-ray machine it is taken off the conveyer. "Do you have a fork in your bag?" the lady asks. I pull out the plastic box, opening it so she can see all my equipment. I write her a note I have a stomach feeding tube and I need this for my medication. This time no tears! I'm angry. In the morning I got through the Sydney screening all right. Other times in Melbourne the people at the x-ray stop my bag and ask to look at my aerosol hairspray. No other security screening at any airport in Australia or New Zealand ask to look at my hairspray. What's wrong in Melbourne? The lady takes my fork to her supervisor who feels the prongs. "They are blunt - it's OK" she says. However, when I get home I replace my metal fork with a plastic one. I don't need these hassles when I travel.

So far I haven't had any problems passing through the x-ray screening with the AFO strapped to my leg. One other time at an airport security x-ray, in Perth, the lady picks me out for random explosives scanning. This has happened to me on several occasions before. I decide to be cheeky "Do I look like a terrorist?" I ask. She doesn't understand me. "It's alright dear" she says, which only serves to make me tearful. It's just so frustrating!

A week or so later I'm back in Perth. The Esplanade Hotel in Fremantle is fully booked so I stay at Rydges Hotel in the Perth central business district. It's a great location and I've stayed here several times. In the week before Christmas last year I was able to do some last minute Christmas shopping. This time I've got a blister on the heel of my left foot and I pop in to the Priceline pharmacy across the road and buy some sticking plasters.

That evening I'm filling my hot water bottle from the just boiled jug of water. I thought I was being careful but the jug is heavy and my left hand is weak. The next thing that I know I'm tipping boiling water down my front! Through the layers of clothing the water hasn't quite reached my skin so I keep filling the hot water bottle. Then suddenly the pain hits me. I screw the stopper on to my hot water bottle and quickly wet a flannel under the cold tap and put it on my stomach. That helps a bit and I sit down waiting for the pain to subside. The scald is worse than I had realised and I fill the flannel with ice cubes and re-apply it to my stomach. The ice has melted and the pain is no better. Next I get a bottle of beer out of the mini bar fridge and press this to the scald. Eventually I feel comfortable enough to get into bed and surprisingly, I sleep quite well.

The scald is right at waistband level, fortunately on the opposite side to the PEG tube. In the morning two huge blisters have formed and there is no way I will be able to do up my trousers without bursting the blisters. Luckily I have my non-stick dressing pads with me. I burst the blisters and the large pad is just the right size to cover the scalded area. Using two of the sticking plasters I bought the afternoon before I can attach the dressing pad to my abdomen. That afternoon back at the Priceline Pharmacy I buy another box of non-stick pads and a roll of Micropore sticking tape. I'm wondering what it is about Perth, as this is the second accident that I've had while I've been there. However, it's fortunate that I was staying at Rydges hotel with the pharmacy right across the road.

I'm away from home for several days each week. The discomfort around the PEG tube has settled down and I'm beginning to wonder how I ever managed without it. Taking medication is so much easier. Similarly, having an adequate fluid intake is no longer a problem. I'm eating breakfast, my usual porridge when I'm at home and bacon, hash browns and poached eggs when I'm away. The hash browns dipped in the egg yolk slip down easily. The bacon is sometimes a little harder to eat depending on how well it is cooked. One morning the rashers were as hard as tough plastic and fused together! I have always loved bacon and now I judge hotels on how well their bacon is cooked! Some hotels are excellent and others serve fatty, cheap mass-cooked bacon that is just awful.

By now I'm used to taking my medication, fluids or Jevity Hi-cal via the tube when I'm at a hospital, in an airport or on the plane. I just get my gear out and do it. It's a matter of having to: my busy lifestyle doesn't leave me any other choice. I usually eat regular food for breakfast and dinner and try and have one tin of Jevity at about 11am and another at 1 or 2pm.

On an early morning flight from Sydney to Christchurch I try to eat the breakfast but I can only manage the bacon. The scrambled egg seems like lots of little round balls of egg and they just won't go down. Next I try the yoghurt but it is too sour and I can't swallow that either, so I give up and have a can of my Jevity and, like Goldilocks, it is just right! When the cabin attendant sees me having a tube feed she stops and asks "Do you have a medical condition that we should know about?" In response I write I travel every week - (I'm) OK. A week later on a flight from Sydney to Auckland the same cabin attendant is on the flight and greets me "Hello again, you're back again, I had you last week. How are you?" No questions this time about my fitness to fly.

A few days earlier on an early afternoon flight from Brisbane to Sydney I have a can of Jevity for lunch. The cabin crew see me as they are serving the lunch and don't say anything to me. Arriving in Sydney in blustery weather the plane lands rather heavily. Having turned up at Brisbane airport with a flexi ticket to get on the next plane going to Sydney I am sitting in the second to last row at the back of the plane. The latch on the drinks trolley can't have been closed properly because as the plane bumps down on to the runway there is an almighty crash behind me and all the little bottles of wine come rolling down the aisle. Some break and others are snatched up by passengers and everyone is laughing.

I seem to be getting by OK phoning from home for a taxi to the airport. The automated answering machine does not understand me and I'm transferred to an operator. Fortunately the computer system displays my address so it is just a matter of me saying "yes" to confirm my address. Although when they ask my destination and I say airport they think I want to go to Enmore! One time it takes me a while to convince one taxi driver that the cab is for me and that I am going to the airport not to Enmore! But once he realises that I have lost my voice he is ever so nice and we chat (me writing responses) and laugh all the way to the airport.

Another time in Christchurch taking a taxi from the hotel to Christchurch Hospital I show the driver my note Christchurch Hospital Main Entrance. A few minutes later while talking on his mobile phone I hear him saying "I'm taking a deaf lady to Christchurch Hospital." I write another note Not deaf Just lost voice. "I'm sorry, my partner's daughter is deaf, she's a really lovely girl" he says. The very next day the same taxi driver takes me from the hotel to the airport. He greets me with a smile "Hello again."

At the beginning of August I attend the 54th Annual Scientific Meeting of the Cardiac Society of Australia and New Zealand (CSANZ) in Canberra, the first that I've attended since I've had the PEG tube. Looking back at last year's CSANZ meeting in Perth I remember thinking *Next year's meeting is in Canberra. I wonder if I will be there? Will I be confined to a wheel chair, unable to talk? Will I even be alive? Well here I am. I can't talk, almost can't eat but I'm still walking and still very much alive!*

Just as I did at the CSANZ conference in Auckland earlier in the year, I stick a note on my conference ID tag: **I've lost my voice. Talk to me** and get on with the business of attending the conference.

I need to take my Jevity at 11 am and 2pm as well as my 5pm Riluzole. In the Convention Centre I just find myself a seat in a corner of the lobby or outside in the sun and get on with it.

The first time, I'm sitting in a corner of the lobby holding up my 50ml syringe full of Jevity when a Sydney-based doctor I haven't seen since 2001 comes and sits opposite me. "Hello, how are you?" he asks. I give an upturned hands wave indicating 'so so' "What's been happening?" he asks pointing to the PEG tube. I struggle to manage to hold the tube and write things down at the same time. Somehow I let him know that I have MND and that I'm living and working in Sydney. I still find it quite distressing telling people who have known me before what's wrong and I can't help a few tears.

There aren't many Kiwis at the conference. I guess most of them went to the conference in Auckland earlier in the year. I manage to catch up with most of the people I know. Some know what's wrong with me and others don't. Later that day I have a chat with an Auckland surgeon I haven't seen since I left Green Lane Hospital. He tells me that his uncle died of MND and asks if he can tell his wife who knows both Mum and me. In the bus going back to the hotel a paediatric cardiologist whom I also haven't seen since I left Green Lane sits in the row behind me. I manage to maintain a conversation with him by writing things down.

On Sunday at lunch time I meet up with a friend from Adelaide. We find a couple of seats in corner and sit down and chat. One of the international speakers comes over and looks at a display right by where we are sitting. Our team at Green Lane worked closely with this doctor for many years. I've had dinner with some of our team at his ranch in North Carolina. I jump up from my seat saying "Hello" and holding out my hand to shake his hand. At the same time I'm pointing to the **I've lost my voice** on my name tag. Initially he doesn't recognize me and I wonder if he thinks that I'm mad! I write I have MND and on second thoughts I write ALS. Later I ask an Auckland colleague to tell him that I'm not mad.

A very well known and respected British cardiologist from Nottingham is another invited speaker at the conference. His work is well known to me - our group at Green Lane worked on many studies with him and my former boss at Green Lane has worked with him on studies in the UK. He doesn't know me but I want to say hello to him. During one of the tea breaks I have an opportunity to say "hello". I point to my name and the **I've lost my voice** on name tag and then write *I've worked with Robin Norris and Harvey White*. Madness or not, I'm familiar with some of his work and if I could speak I would love to have a chat to him about his thoughts on obtaining informed consent for participation in clinical trials during acute myocardial infarction.

I attend the conference sessions but on the social side I miss the welcome reception, the conference dinner and the 5pm wine and poster sessions. I'm too tired and also I can't drink wine anymore. My friend from Adelaide said I should just put it down the tube! But it's not the same. Strangely I don't miss wine or the food I can't eat.

The hotel I'm staying in turns out to be the Australian International Hotel Training School. On the first night when I ask for room service dinner the man at reception says the restaurant is closed for two weeks because they don't have a chef! He gives me a Thai take away menu! I tell him that *I have a stomach feeding tube and can only eat soft food. I chose to stay here because on the internet it said that you have a restaurant*. The duty manager comes along. "We have a function here tonight and can get you something to eat" he says and he offers to make me something in the kitchen over the weekend. The meal on Friday night is the best hotel meal I've had in a long time; steamed fish with mashed potato and a lovely orange sauce. The following night they cook me braised lamb shank which is nice. But on Sunday, given the choice of fish and mashed potato or chicken I choose fish. The fish and mashed potato are cold and not very nice at all. I can only eat a little and end up raiding the mini bar and nibbling on a bar of chocolate. However, the staff at the hotel are very kind and try their best to accommodate me.

13
Baltic Cruise - August 2006

My mother has asked me to accompany her on a 14 day Baltic cruise in August. Initially, before the PEG insertion, I have misgivings about the trip, being unsure how I will manage the PEG tube which I will have by then. I'm still not sure when I'm in Auckland. On Saturday evening we have dinner with my sister Jenni, her husband Francis and a couple of other friends. Jenni has friends who have been on a similar cruise. Like me they went on the cruise at short notice and thoroughly enjoyed it. Of course Jenni is right, I travel all the time for my job, I'm no stranger to airports and planes or in fact, cruise ships. This ship, the *Regatta*, is a sister ship to the *Insignia* which Mum and I were on in January 2005 on our South American cruise, and Kevin and I were on an identical ship in January 2006 on our Tahitian cruise.

"You'll never get another chance. You should go" Jenni says. And of course she is right. When I get back to Sydney I start organising flights from Sydney to London returning from Stockholm to Sydney.

Initially I book a return economy trip Sydney to London returning Stockholm to Sydney. I have plans to use my frequent flyer points to upgrade to business class. I realise that I have enough points to upgrade only one way, and this is not guaranteed as upgrades are issued only on departure. I start to think about purchasing business class tickets. I'll be flying approximately 24 hours each way. I'll need to have several tube feeds of Jevity, take my medication and take fluids via the tube. I think that

I will probably get better assistance from the business class cabin crew.

I'm still thinking about it when I return from Perth on a Boeing 747. I have an aisle seat in the forward economy cabin. This is a good seat and I won't get anything better in economy on my trip to London. Before the plane has even left the gate in Perth the pilot announces "I'm sorry about the delay, folks, we have a passenger who won't be travelling with us and we need to off load her luggage." Time goes on, paramedics come on to the plane and walk towards the back of the plane. Then another announcement: "You have probably seen the activity. A passenger has been hit on the head by falling luggage and she is being taken to hospital." While all this is going on two little children in the seats behind me keep up a constant high pitched chatter, kicking the back of my seat at the same time. I wonder why their parents aren't doing more to keep them quiet. Several times I have to stop myself getting up and going "Sush!!" to them. The man sitting next to me has overpowering aftershave on and it's all getting very frustrating. Eventually after about an hour on the ground we are finally on our way to Sydney and my mind is made up. I'll buy business class seats to London and back!

I've worked very hard for the savings that I have. Since I've been living and working in Sydney, despite paying rent in Sydney and for some of the time also paying half of our mortgage in Auckland, I have been saving regularly. I won't now be using my savings for my retirement and where I'm going I can't take it with me. This is sure to be my last trip to Europe, I'll treat myself.

Mum mentioned to me in a letter that "it would be helpful to have your medical information to give to the ship so they have lots of suitable food." I told her not to worry because there would be plenty of regular food that I could eat and I always travel with my medical information. I thought nothing more of it.

Next thing I know I get an email from Kevin entitled URGENT:

> The cruise MUST have a signed letter from your Doctor to say you are fit to travel.

I'm upset by this. I know I'm fit to travel, I do it every week! Unless I try to speak, no one knows that there is anything wrong with me. Feeling angry about the inconvenience of this I send an email to the travel agent in Auckland who is handling the cruise reservation.

> I have received an urgent request from my husband Kevin to contact you regarding my fitness to travel.
> Firstly let me explain my situation.
> I live alone in Sydney and work full time as a clinical research associate. My work involves travel by air to major cities in Australia and New Zealand on a weekly basis. For example I spent 3 days in Perth last week and will spend 4 days in Brisbane this week, followed by Christchurch and then Auckland the following 2 weeks.
>
> I was diagnosed with motor neurone disease in August 2004 and immediately commenced taking medication that slows the progression of the disease. This medication is not available in New Zealand hence my decision to remain in Australia. I have lost the ability to speak and have a stomach feeding tube for some feeds, all medication and most fluids. I will be bringing all the enteral feeds (in tins) that I need with me. I will also be bringing documentation for the enteral feeds should there be any problems with customs. I have taken this product with me on my trips to NZ without problems. The cruise ship WILL NOT NEED TO SUPPLY ANYTHING.
>
> In the past 18 months I have been on 2 other cruises, one in South America with Mum and one in Tahiti with my husband; both were entirely trouble free. I have no concerns about my ability to manage my condition while I am away.
>
> I am fully mobile and do not require any assistance.
>
> I will be travelling to/from Europe with Qantas ex Sydney.

I have booked business class seats and expect to have a trouble free trip.

I am in the process of obtaining a doctor's declaration for medical insurance to cover an existing condition. I have an appointment with one of my specialists on 17 July. I always travel with my medical documents that explain my condition and medication. I will have these with me on the cruise.

Please contact me by email should you require further information or have any questions. I am in the office today, however for the rest of this week while I am in Brisbane I will only be checking emails morning and evening.

Kind regards,
Barbara Williams.

I am reasonably satisfied with the reply that I get from the NZ travel agent:

Thank you for your email.
May I explain that for any passengers with medical problems it is essential we pass this on to the airline or as in this case the cruise line for the protection of both parties which I did on information received from your Mother. The cruise line has asked for a signed letter from your doctor confirming your fitness to travel before they will accept this booking. I am sure from what both you and your Mother have said there should not be a problem.
I have forwarded your email to the cruise line in the hopes that this will satisfy them.

However the next day another email arrives:

Hi Barbara,

Sorry about this but have received the following reply from the cruise line. Can you email your doctor and ask him to EMAIL and FAX a letter to me so I can get this processed.

Again I am sorry to put you through this but it is a normal requirement.

He includes the email from the cruise line's New Zealand agent:

> Hi there,
>
> I have been advised the following from the cruise line:
> Sorry we will not accept her as a passenger until she can provide us with the letter.
>
> As per our requirements we will require a "Fit to travel letter" typed and signed by passenger's doctor, and an indication from doctor regarding what her actual needs would be onboard. Once they have this they have advised they will be able to give an appropriate response.

By now I'm quite cross. I'm sure Mum thought she was being helpful but this is so unnecessary. I know very well that I'll be fitter than a lot of elderly people and obese people who will be on the cruise. I'm in Brisbane and won't be back in Sydney until late Friday afternoon. I email Margie and ask her advice. Fortunately I get a prompt response from Margie suggesting that I draft a letter that my Neurologist can sign. The letter is duly faxed to the NZ travel agent.

> I have just received the letter thanks. Have forwarded it on and hopefully we will have a favourable reply by Monday.

There is no email from the travel agent on Monday morning so I send another email to him:

> Have you had a response from the cruise company yet? I'm seeing another specialist today and could get an additional letter of support from him if necessary.

Fortunately before I leave for my doctor's appointment an email arrives from the travel agent:

> Hi Barbara,
> Great news have just had confirmation of your booking.

I have an annual travel insurance policy for my work but it does not cover existing medical conditions. I email the Sydney travel agent who is handling my plane reservations:

> I wonder if you could give me a quote for travel insurance to cover the time period. I have the annual global travel insurance cover that is valid thru to December 2006. However, it does not cover existing medical conditions. I have motor neurone disease which is not covered by that policy. I am still mobile and independent, however I have lost my voice. To date I have not had any medical problems while I have been travelling. I guess I'll need to get some sort of a medical certificate for the travel insurance. Over the past 18 months I have travelled in South America and French Polynesia, with the travel insurance as above, and been trouble free.

The travel agent sends me an application form for travel insurance that covers some pre-existing medical conditions. There are two forms, one for me to complete and a medical declaration for my doctor to complete.

There are two clauses that I'm unsure about:

- Have you been given a terminal prognosis for any condition with a life expectancy of less than 24 months?
- Any condition for which you have been hospitalised in the 24 months prior to purchasing your policy.

None of my doctors has given me any indication of my life expectancy. From all of my reading, I understand that the rate of progression of MND is different in each person. If Mum had asked me last Christmas if I would like to go on this cruise with her in August, I would have said "I don't know if I will still be well enough in August" just as I was reluctant to commit myself to going to somewhere in Europe last Christmas. For more than one year or so, I haven't planned anything work-wise or for leisure more than about three or four weeks in advance. In May last year I renewed my gym membership for three months, only extending it to a full year once the first three months were up and I've done the same this year. In June last year I had to renew the lease on my apartment. I had the choice of renewing it for six or twelve months. I renewed it for six, knowing full well that I was leaving myself open to another rent rise when the term of the lease was up. Fortunately that hasn't happened and I'm still in the apartment, lease expired and no increase in rent - so far.

At a medical consultation I ask the doctor to complete the medical declaration page of the insurance for me. He does this willingly. Later that day I'm making a photocopy of the insurance form before I mail it. I'm watching the pages pass through the automatic feed when the photocopier jams and the pages are gobbled up. Feeling a sense of doom, I wonder what to do. I can't submit these crumpled pages. I duly print out another set of forms, I fill in my declaration and mail the forms to the doctor asking if he would complete another medical declaration for me and mail it in the stamped addressed envelope to the travel agent. I continue with my busy schedule of work and travel.

Two weeks before I'm due to fly to London I'm in Auckland for work. Kevin has the flu and so not wanting to catch it from him, I stay with Mum in the apartment that she moved to earlier this year. The apartment building is about 100 metre walk to Hurstmere Road and the same distance to Takapuna beach. On Friday and Saturday afternoons we walk along Takapuna beach to the southern end and sit on a rock in the sun talking and watching the activities on the beach and looking at the magnificent view of Rangitoto, the Hauraki Gulf, Whangaparaoa Peninsula, the Coromandel Ranges and Great Barrier Island in the distance. Watching dogs chasing seagulls along the beach, children playing in rock pools - it's just idyllic. I've had a really special weekend at Mum's.

I love the beaches of Auckland's Hauraki Gulf. I've grown up with these beaches almost in my back yard. Some of my earliest memories are of looking out at Rangitoto from my first storey bedroom window at our North Shore home. I went to kindergarten across the road from Narrow Neck Beach and our teachers often took us over to the beach to walk or play. I was born in the old Narrow Neck camp hospital. My passport records my place of birth as Narrow Neck. On my arrival in New Zealand immigration officials often ask "Where is Narrow Neck?" In later years when we lived in Kohimarama and then Wellington we spent our school holidays on the beach at Hatfield's and Orewa beaches. Summer and winter we spent time at the beach, playing in the sand, climbing in the Pohutukawa trees, searching for shrimps in the rock pools, fishing for tiddlers off the rocks and of course swimming. Even in the winter holidays if there was a storm and big waves at Hatfield's beach we would take our polystyrene surfboards down to the beach and ride in on the surf. If the waves were too choppy for that we just jumped about in the 'soap suds' having fun.

A week before I'm due to travel to London, I email the travel agent to see how my insurance application is getting on. She replies:

> I haven't received any insurance forms for you as yet

Luckily I'm seeing another doctor that afternoon and I ask him to complete the medical declaration for me. This he does but I get the feeling that he doesn't like my chances of being successful with the company covering my existing condition. I mail off the forms and two days later I get a response from the travel agent:

> I've had a response from the Medical Assessment Board and they have said that they won't cover you for any claims arising from the PEG tube insertion and the Motor Neurone Disease.
>
> They will offer you the standard cover for any other claims which is $175.00 for the duration of your trip.

I don't need standard cover; I have an annual business travel insurance policy and I reply:

> I have an annual business travel insurance policy that covers everything except existing conditions. What I was wanting was the additional cover. Quite frankly I think travel insurance companies are unfair. They are quite happy to collect the money from people but won't take a slight risk that they might have to pay out. In the 2 years that I have had MND I have travelled extensively and not made one claim for illness or anything else.

The travel agent advises me that I can appeal the decision not to cover any claims arising from MND or the PEG insertion. It's worth a try so I email the insurance company:

I wish to appeal the decision not to cover any claims arising from my existing medical condition of Motor Neurone disease and the PEG tube insertion.

In my work as a clinical research associate I travel to capital cities within Australia and New Zealand on an almost weekly basis. In addition since I have been diagnosed with Motor Neurone Disease I have travelled within South America (Jan 2005) and Tahiti (Jan 2006) and I never had one insurance claim for illness or otherwise.

The PEG tube insertion has been uncomplicated and has improved my overall condition in that I now take all medication and most fluids via the tube, thus minimising the risk of choking or inhaling fluid.

I have also lost my voice BUT this does NOT stop me travelling, working full time and living independently.
In my opinion I am at most risk of the following:

1) falling over: I have an AFO ankle foot brace which has stabilised my left foot. I will be wearing this at all times and I have also purchased a walking stick which I will use for extra stability. Before getting the AFO I had 2 falls which did not result in the need for medical treatment. Since getting the AFO I have not fallen.

2) a respiratory infection, which in itself is not attributable to MND. This winter I have had influenza and pneumoccal vaccinations and have not had a single winter respiratory illness or cold despite almost weekly airline travel.

As indicated on my application form, I have a current annual global business travel insurance policy, however it does not cover existing medical conditions.

For further information you may contact the Motor Neurone Disease nurse coordinator (name and mobile phone number supplied). She has access to my medical records and can put you in touch with my neurologist if necessary.

My date of departure is this Sunday Aug 13 so I would appreciate a quick decision .

In the meantime, I hear breaking news on the radio that a terrorist plot to blow up transatlantic airliners has been uncovered in Britain. I learn that security procedures have been tightened for passengers on flights to Britain and the US and carry-on luggage is to be placed in plastic bags.

I email the travel agent and in her response she includes the new carry-on restrictions:

> Passengers will be allowed to take through the airport security search point, in a single (ideally transparent) plastic carrier bag, only the following items. Nothing may be carried in pockets:
>
> - pocket size wallets and pocket size purses plus contents (eg money, credit cards, identity cards etc (no handbags) travel documents essential for the journey (for example passports and travel tickets).
> - prescription medicines and medical items sufficient and essential for the flight (e.g. diabetic kit), except in liquid form unless verified as authentic.
> - spectacles and sunglasses, without cases; contact lens holders, without bottles of solution.
> - for those travelling with an infant: baby food, milk (the contents of each bottle must be tasted by the accompanying passenger) and sanitary items sufficient and essential for the flight (nappies, wipes, creams and nappy disposal bags).
> - female sanitary items sufficient and essential for the flight, if unboxed (e.g. tampons, pads, towels and wipes) tissues (unboxed) and/or handkerchiefs.
> - keys (but no electrical key fobs).
>
> All passengers will be hand searched, and their footwear and all the items they are carrying will be x-ray screened.
>
> Pushchairs and walking aids will be x-ray screened, and only airport-provided wheelchairs will be allowed to pass through the screening point.

At the end of the email she also tells me that the travel insurance company has again declined the coverage for MND and the PEG tube. This makes me very angry. I feel it is discrimination. Perhaps my frank email has only reinforced their decision, but at least I've been honest. I don't think that the company has even taken the time to consider my case as an individual, to weigh up my individual risk, but right now I don't have time to pursue it. Time will tell.

I've packed 36 cans of Jevity for my trip in a photocopy box. I've stuck a label off a can and a typed note with my name and destination etc on the top of the box. The dietician has sent me a letter verifying my need for the product - but he emailed it on plain paper with no signature. I think in the current environment of increased airline security an unsigned letter on plain paper might raise security questions, so I email the dietician asking for a signed letter on hospital letterhead. I'm about to take a trip over the road to the hospital to see if I can find the dietician when I get an email saying that he will put five copies of a signed letter in my letterbox.

I tape one copy of the letter in a plastic cover to the outside of the box and put another copy inside the box. I will take a couple of copies with me in my carry-on luggage and hope that this will satisfy both the security inspections and the agricultural and customs inspections. I'm prepared to pull up my shirt and show them my PEG tube if need be to prove my need for the Jevity and other equipment that I will need to carry on to the plane. Again time will tell.

I wonder if the terrorists had plans for a repeat attack on 11 September? Ironically my mother and I were travelling in Sweden and Norway at the time of the 9/11 tragedy in 2001. I had been in Stockholm attending the Annual Congress of the European Society of Cardiology where I had a poster presentation of the results of my study on informed consent. This is the study that was subsequently published in the *Lancet.*

On Saturday before my Sunday departure to London I'm busily sorting out clear plastic bags for my carry-on luggage when my mobile phone rings. "Uloooo" is my slurred greeting. "Mrs. Williams?" asks the male voice. "Uloooo" I repeat and the line goes dead. Then my landline phone rings. It's a man from Qantas. He explains that there are no restrictions on carry-on luggage for my flight to London tomorrow but that I'll need to check if there are still restrictions for my homeward flight from London. I'll take a selection of plastic bags in my luggage in case I need them on the way home.

Sunday comes and I'm all packed and ready to go. I take the rubbish down to the garbage room and in the elevator coming back up to the sixth floor I meet my neighbour, Phil. Phil knows that I've lost my voice and some time ago he said "Let me know if you need any help." I scribble a quick note *I'm going to London this afternoon. Could you please phone a taxi for me and help me with my luggage?* Phil kindly calls a taxi for me and takes my heavy case and box of cans down to the taxi and I'm on my way.

I have no problems checking in or going through the security x-ray screening and I have an uneventful flight via Bangkok to London's Heathrow airport. On arrival at Heathrow I wait at the baggage carousel for what seems like ages for my luggage to arrive. Having business class tags does not mean that it arrives any faster. Just as I'm beginning to wonder if my luggage is lost or worse, in these times of heightened airline security, has been off loaded because of my tins of Jevity, I see my box of Jevity on the carousel followed by my suitcase.

I pass through the green lane at the customs checkpoint without any problems. My box of Jevity is sitting on top of my suitcase on the luggage trolley and no one even asks me about the contents. In the arrivals hall I can't see the Oceania Cruises representative. After waiting for ages I write **OCEANIA** on a piece of paper and wander around holding it up. Just as I am beginning to despair I see a lady with an official **OCEANIA** sign. She is waiting for me and fairly soon we are on our way to the Holland Park Hilton Hotel.

Mum is arriving later in the morning so I go out for a walk to Notting Hill Gate. It's a dull overcast mid-August day and as I'm walking there are a few spits of rain. At Notting Hill Gate I check the location of the tube station. I have pre-purchased (on the internet) tickets for a tour of Buckingham Palace and as soon as Mum arrives we head off to the tube station. I realise that I have left my walking stick in the hotel room but we are in a hurry and I don't go back for it. As I'm walking along the road the strapping on my AFO starts to slip and the upper bar on the AFO pops out of the strap. I stop and refasten the AFO. This happens several more times during the course of the afternoon however we press on, anxious to reach Buckingham Palace before admissions to the tour of the palace close.

We take the tube from Notting Hill Gate to Green Park and then walk through the park to the palace. Having our pre-paid tickets means that we can miss the queues of people waiting to buy tickets and we are soon in a holding area waiting to be let into the palace.

We enter through the Ambassador's entrance and although we pass through the various state rooms fairly quickly we have time to take in the furnishings, paintings and gold embossing. Mum talks about the times that she has been in the palace at official functions and she points out the rooms that she has been in. While appreciating the magnificence of the rooms I think that for the Royal Family it must be like living in a museum, although I do realise that these rooms aren't actually 'lived in'.

As we pass through the room where the investitures are held I ask Mum if this is where Dad was knighted. "No, that was at Windsor Castle" Mum replies.

As part of the Queen's 80th birthday celebrations there is a display of some of the Queen's evening dresses and her private jewelry. This is the highlight of our visit. The dresses are grouped in colours. The dresses on display include some of her early dresses and it's interesting to see how the dress styles have changed over the years. Unchanged, however, is the magnificent beading on all of the dresses. This room is packed with people and Mum and I shuffle past all the displays sticking close to the barriers so that we can see and also read the information about each dress. Several were worn on visits to New Zealand or at Commonwealth Heads of Government meetings that Mum and Dad attended. The jewelry is wonderful too. I recognize several of the pieces including the choker that the Princess of Wales wore once as a headband. I remember several years ago there was an exhibition in Wellington of the Princess of Wales' evening dresses. Mum and I flew from Auckland to Wellington for the day to see the exhibition. The striking thing about both the Queen's and Diana's dresses is the magnificent bead work.

The Queen's Orders (medals) are displayed in the adjoining ball room. As we are just starting to look at these an official tells us that we all have to leave the room for security reasons. He says that we can come back later but it's now 5pm and we decide to return to the hotel.

We leave the palace through the garden and find ourselves on the street nearer to Hyde Park than to Green Park. A quick look at my map and I decide we should to go to Hyde Park tube station. We walk in the general direction of Hyde Park and soon I recognize the entrance to the tube station. On my first visit to London, attending a meeting in 1993, I stayed at the Park Lane Hilton Hotel and Hyde Park was the nearest tube station. We need to change trains twice to reach Notting Hill Gate but apart from the walking involved it's fairly easy.

Travelling around London on the tube is so easy. London is great! *Why didn't I come to London again for a few days while I was fairly fit?* I wonder. I would like to come back again for a few days soon.

I have needed to stop several times to re-adjust my AFO while we were out and back at the hotel I examine the strapping. I immediately see the problem. Some of the stitching has pulled apart and there is nothing to stop the strapping from pulling away from the upper support of the AFO. Fortunately I have a small sewing kit with me and Mum stitches it up for me as my hands don't work well enough any more for sewing. The strapping is still slipping though, and it needs something to stop it riding up. I cut one of my knee high stockings into strips. I wind the strips around the strapping and the bar and ask Mum to tie the knots. Again my hands don't work well enough for knot tying. This does the trick and for the rest of the trip I have no more trouble with the AFO.

In the morning we are up fairly early and shortly after 8am we are waiting in the hotel lobby for the bus to take us to Dover. When the bus arrives I wander out to make sure my box of Jevity is safe. I write a note to the man loading the luggage to make sure my box is not damaged pointing to the box at the same time. He picks up the box and places it on a seat in the bus, strapping it in with the seat belt. "Hop in the bus" he says. Mum and I are first in the bus and we choose the front seats so we can have an unobstructed view as we drive to Dover.

Soon we are on our way passing firstly through the leafy streets of Kensington. Next we pass Harrods, Hyde Park corner where we entered the tube station yesterday, and drive past the back garden wall of Buckingham Palace. We pass Westminster, Big Ben, Downing Street, Tower Bridge and the Tower of London and on into the East End. I note the difference between the grand town houses in Kensington and the housing blocks in the east of London.

Again I wonder *Why haven't I come back to London sooner?* During the 1990s I have had several fleeting visits to London, the first in 1993 for a meeting at the Park Lane Hilton and on several other occasions passing through London on the way to or from meetings in other European cities. I have always packed a lot into these visits and managed to see a surprising number of the 'must see' London attractions but I've never been in London for longer than three days at any one time.

On the drive through the English countryside I note with interest the number of large European trucks (identified by the driver sitting on the left hand side of the truck) driving towards London having come over on one of the roll-on roll-off ferries.

Arriving in Dover I supervise the unloading of my box of Jevity. It is put into a wheelchair and a man kindly pushes it along with us as we check in for the cruise and pass through the x-ray security screening. He arranges for someone from the ship to accompany us to our cabin carrying the box. The box of Jevity is safely installed in our cabin, undamaged and unchallenged. So far so good!

With only 600 passengers the *Regatta* is small enough to be friendly and Mum and I immediately feel at home on the ship. At the purser's desk I cash a traveller's cheque. I sign the cheque and hand it to the lady. She looks at it and says "Can you please sign again on the back?" I do this and then she takes the cheque to the Purser and they have a discussion. The problem is that my signatures are not identical! I write her a note My hand is paralyzed. "We will have a problem when we bank it" she says. However, she cashes the cheque and hands me 50 Euros.

Overnight we sail to Zeebrugge, the scene of the 1987 disaster where the roll-on roll-off ferry *Herald of Free Enterprise* capsized 90 seconds out of port on a crossing from Belgium to Britain.

Having both previously been to Brussels, Mum and I choose the tour to Brugges, a lovely medieval town with narrow cobbled streets and peaceful canals. The tour is predominantly a walking tour and even though the activity level has been designated as strenuous, with my walking stick I have no trouble keeping up with everyone. We visit the Church of Notre Dame where we see a Michelangelo statue of Mary and the Holy Child. The tour includes a 30 minute canal boat ride. The canals are quite serene and peaceful but don't look at the water - it's dirty and there is algae in it. At the end of the tour we are given 30 minutes for shopping. Mum goes into the lace and tapestry shop and I put my backpack on an outside café table and have a tin of Jevity via the tube.

In the evening, as we sail out of Zeebrugge, Mum and I are in the Grand Dining Room seated at a table for two by the window having dinner. Out in the North Sea the shipping lanes are marked with buoys and there is two-way shipping traffic just like a highway. We watch with interest as an eclectic mix of freighters and ferries pass.

The following day we are in Amsterdam. This is my third visit to the Netherlands and Mum and I have both been to Amsterdam. This time we go on a tour to the fishing hamlet of Marken. There are quaint green and white clapboard houses that date back to the 13th century. As we wander through the winding lanes between the houses our guide points out the peg-less washing hanging on the washing lines. Two strings of twisted line are strung up and the washing is attached by pushing the corners of the garments between the twists. *I couldn't do this,* I think, *I can barely manage pegs.*

Then we drive to the 14th century town of Volendam where we see narrow canals and drawbridges. The town is on the shores of the former Zuiderzee. When the Zuiderzee was closed off from the North Sea the salt water inlet changed into a fresh water lake and it is now called Lake Usselmeer. I remember seeing the modern day windmills on the barrier dyke between the North Sea and the lake during the Easter weekend that I spent in the Netherlands in 2000. Driving back to the Regatta through the Dutch countryside our guide explains how dykes are built and how canals and pumps are used to drain the land and to keep it dry. She explains that the polders are below sea level and points out canals where the water level is well above the level of the land.

Overnight we sail northwards and in the morning the *Regatta* enters the Kiel Canal. The canal is 98 km long and runs through the Schleswig-Holstein region of Germany, connecting the North Sea with the Baltic Sea. There are locks at each end of the canal to minimize tidal variation. Along with other ships we wait our turn to enter the lock and pass into the canal. After the early starts of the last few days we enjoy a sleep in and a leisurely breakfast in the Grand Dining Room.

During the day we sit in the Horizons Lounge high above the bow of the ship and watch as we sail through the countryside. Most of the land surrounding the canal is farmland. There are people walking or cycling along paths beside the canal, people fishing and occasionally a road or rail bridge or a ferry crossing the canal. It's reminiscent of scenes in the Gota canal between Stockholm and Gothenberg in Sweden where in September 2001 Mum and I spent four days on the Gota canal cruise.

An American lady who is sitting next to me starts asking me questions. I write her a quick note *I've lost my voice*. "You are very brave to be travelling. Are you on your own?" she asks. *No this is my mother.* I answer and point to Mum who sitting next to me on the other side. She starts talking to Mum and after a while, feeling a little left out of the conversation, I get up and move away.

Later that evening we have dinner with an American couple who I discover are involved in clinical trials. He is a doctor and his wife a study coordinator. We have a great conversation, with me writing things down. Another night the man sitting next to me has worked for an American pharmaceutical company before he retired. Again we have things in common and have a good conversation.

By now the waiters know me. I write down what I want, starting off: *I've lost my voice. I also have trouble swallowing and I'm very slow. I would like to have my meal first up while mother is having soup.* After the first couple of nights I realise that the vegetables are too difficult to eat. Even the mashed potato is too slushy and seeps out through my lips. I can manage the french fries because I can use my fingers to place them directly between my molars and chew them. Similarly in the morning I can place the crispy bacon directly in the right place. So I have crispy bacon, hash browns and poached or scrambled eggs for breakfast every morning. At home I have porridge for breakfast but the porridge on the ship is too runny and like the mashed potato it seeps out through my lips. Most of my trouble with eating is manoeuvreing the food around in my mouth. I'm having two cans of Jevity in the middle of the day so I'm still getting all the vitamins and minerals that I need.

The next morning we arrive at Warnemünde in the former East Germany. We choose a tour of the nearby Hanseatic city of Rostock. Our guide is a young lady who has lived through the reunification of Germany and the change-over of currency to the Euro. "We have had the value of our money cut in half twice, once changing to the German Mark and then again changing to the Euro" she says. She points out the apartment where she lived as a child. It's in a typical Soviet-type block of residential apartments. "We were lucky," she says. "We had a small balcony." Most of the apartments don't have a balcony and most apartment buildings are five storeys high. "There are no elevators in five storey apartment buildings," she explains. Her mother, who worked in a local factory, would take her by tram to daycare and then board another tram to go to work. Our guide had studied engineering at the Rostock University which she said is the oldest university in Northern Europe. When the group visits a brewery for beer tasting Mum and I wait outside. I can no longer swallow beer and Mum didn't want any. Standing outside in the car park I have a can of Jevity and Mum wanders around.

In the afternoon we go for a walk in Warnemünde. We walk out along the breakwater between the port and the beach. Warnemünde is a Baltic seaside resort and the beach is crowded with people lying in the sun - it seems to be the German Rivera.

Sailing into Copenhagen the following morning I watch as we pass 20 or more windmills standing in a line out in the harbour. Later I learn that 30% of Denmark's power is generated by windmills. All the way along the coasts of Belgium, the Netherlands and in the Kiel canal we have seen windmills. From a distance they are silent, graceful and somehow relaxing. Yet in Sydney there has been opposition to power generation with windmills. I can't understand why.

Mum has been to Copenhagen before so instead of a city tour we visit the castles of North Zealand. We drive through the countryside for about one hour passing impressive homes and lovely beaches on the way to the Fredriksborg Castle. Apparently this is the castle where Shakespeare's Hamlet is set although it seems that Shakespeare never actually visited the castle himself. The castle stands at the top of a small hill overlooking the strait of water between Denmark and Sweden and although there is misty drizzle, we can see Sweden 5km away. The narrow spiral stone staircases in the castle are a bit of a challenge for me, particularly going up, but aided by my walking stick I manage without any mishaps. It is Sunday and we aren't able to visit the castle's chapel as it serves as the town of Hilleroed's church and a service is in progress. The chapel is supposed to contain the world's oldest organ that is still in use.

In the town we pass the ferry terminal and learn that it's only a 20 minute trip to Sweden. Because of high taxation in Sweden, Danish beer is cheaper and Swedes come over on the ferry to buy cheap beer which is sold from liquor outlets on the pier.

We stop to take photos at Fredensbourg Palace which is the Danish Royal Family's summer residence but of course we can't go inside. The drive back to the ship takes a different route and we pass farmland with horses grazing and learn that Denmark has the highest ratio of horses per head of population, however we don't learn what the horses are used for. Perhaps they are race horses or dressage and jumping but we don't pass any training tracks. We pass fields of small fir trees and learn that they are grown for export as Christmas trees. We also learn that car registration in Denmark is 200% of the purchase price of the car. Presumably this is a one off payment. I guess that's one way to encourage people to use public transport!

We have lunch on the ship and then go out for a walk to find the Little Mermaid statue. As we walk along the foreshore we notice a foul smell. It smells like sewage. We had also noticed a similar smell by the beach and port at Warnemünde. In Copenhagen the water in the boat harbour is covered by a yucky floating mass of a yellowy greenish substance. Perhaps this is the source of the smell.

I wonder if it is algae or sewage. We find the Little Mermaid statue, take photos and walk back to the pier. The pier is lined with factory outlet shops so we wander along looking in the shops. I buy two bottles of Coke but at €3 per 0.5L bottle it's rather expensive and certainly not factory shop prices.

Again we are in the Grand Dining Room at a table for two by the window having dinner as we sail out of Copenhagen. Again we sail past the windmills rising from the water and a little later in the distance we see the outline of the bridge linking Denmark and Sweden.

Next morning we are having breakfast as the *Regatta* sails in to Gdansk, Poland. We have chosen to go on a tour to the former concentration camp at Stutthof. As we leave the ship our passports are stamped by the Polish customs authorities. This is the first time that we have had to show our passports since entering Europe.

As we drive out of the port area our guide talks to us about the ship building industry in Gdansk. He talks with great pride of Lech Walesa and Solidarity. Our guide has worked in the ship building industry and was involved with Solidarity. He says that the three best things that have happened in Poland are 1) joining Nato, 2) Solidarity, 3) the Polish Pope. However, I can see that Poland still has a long way to go. We drive past run-down buildings, un-cut grass, and much of what we see has a tired neglected look about it. The guide mentions how times have been tough and that lots of professional people have left the country. In particular, he mentions that lots of doctors and nurses have left.

We drive into the countryside passing newly harvested fields. It is flat delta land like the Netherlands. Our guide continues to talk to us as we drive along. He tells us that before he was born his parents had been interned in a concentration camp during the war. He doesn't tell us why they were interned but they both survived. Our guide is surprisingly knowledgeable and has a philosophical outlook on things. Both our German guide and this Polish guide seem to be surprisingly well adjusted despite their difficult upbringings in the communist system. Those of us who have grown up in post-war comfort, in first world countries, take so much for granted.

Arriving at Stutthof we firstly watch a short video that outlines the history of the camp. Built in 1939 it is the first concentration camp to be built outside Germany. Initially there were eight barracks for inmates and a large brick house for the SS officers. Later 30 more barracks were added and the gas chamber and crematorium were added in 1943. The camp was liberated in 1945. The tour is listed as easy activity, short walking and some steps. However, I find it difficult to keep up with the fast walking pace.

The shipboard presentation of this tour mentioned that it could be emotionally challenging and was not a tour for everyone. I have an understanding of what occurred in the concentration camps, I've read Michener's novel *Poland*, seen the movie *Schindler's List* and visited Anne Frank's house in Amsterdam. I find this visit to be very interesting but not particularly disturbing. Maybe this is because of the ongoing commentary from our guide or maybe it was the museum-like presentation of the camp. That's not to say that I deny what happened here or that I, in any way, condone or excuse it. I do not. My lasting impression is that it is now a peaceful place in the countryside and a memorial to those who died there. Back on the ship Mum and I speak to an American couple we had met a few days earlier at dinner. The man, whom we think is Jewish, says that he couldn't have gone there because having previously visited holocaust museums he would have found it too distressing.

Before we return to the ship we visit the old town of Gdansk. It's another Hanseatic town. We have a sense of déjà vu as the Hanseatic architecture looks the same here as in the other Hanseatic towns that we visited. Again I have trouble keeping up with the fast walking pace on the cobble stones. We visit the medieval St Mary's Church and I think that everything inside the church needs a good polish to make it shine. Before we entered the church the sky had been looking ominous and when we go back outside it is pouring with rain. Neither Mum nor I have raincoats or umbrellas so we go back into the church to wait until the rain stops. We have about 45 minutes before we need to be back at the meeting place.

We venture out during a break in the rain and head off in what we think is the right direction. The rain starts again and we shelter under a café umbrella in a deserted street café. There is no let up in the rain and I write Mum a note *We had better get going in case we are lost*. So off we go. We get to the end of the street and I don't see anything familiar. We are lost. We shelter in the entrance to a shopping arcade and I ask Mum to ask a couple of young guys how to get to the Golden Gate. She points to it on our map. The guys laugh and say "Italia." They are not locals. However they point us in the right direction, back the way we came and off we hurry in the rain. Luckily we catch sight of some other people on our tour and we follow them. We get back to the meeting point at the Golden Gate with about five minutes to spare. My problem is twofold 1) I can't speak to people to ask for help and 2) I can't walk fast enough to get to a destination quickly if I'm lost.

After Gdansk we have a day at sea sailing to Helsinki. It's nice to have a relaxing day. We have a leisurely breakfast in the Grand Dining Room. We book the remainder of our shore trips, read our books and attend a lecture on Catherine the Great given by an American emeritus professor of art history. Having only just seen a Sunday night T.V. series on Catherine the Great I am already a fan of hers and keen to visit her palace in St Petersburg. The lecturer says that Catherine is one of his 'heroes.' Regardless of her somewhat unconventional morals and extravagant expenditure she did a lot for Russia. She improved agricultural methods, developed mining and several manufacturing industries, abolished export duties to encourage exports, developed town plans, improved education and health care, built up a huge Imperial art collection and so the list goes on. Her achievements are even more remarkable because she was a woman and born a German not a Russian.

For a change we choose a harbour cruise in Helsinki. We start off sitting outside on the upper deck but pretty soon it is too cold and we go inside. As the ice age retreated the sea invaded and Helsinki harbour is a maze of islands, some quite large and populated with vegetation and houses. Others are just small barren smooth rocks sticking out of the water. The port is iced in for about 100 days during winter. Our guide says that this provides opportunities to skate or ski from one island to another or even to drive a car over the ice.

We pass all sizes of houses on the islands, small houses, large luxurious houses and a few apartment buildings. Most of the houses have a small building housing a sauna at the water's edge. The idea is that you hop in the water first, through a hole in the ice in winter and then straight into the sauna. Our tour guide has a husky voice. She says that polluted air from Russia has hung over the city for the past three days. Apparently a hundred or so people were hospitalised with respiratory problems. I guess today's brisk wind has blown the pollution away because the air is OK now.

On the boat trip everyone is served morning tea and cake. I have a tin of Jevity. When we get back to the pier we wander through the open-air market. I see some lovely fur hats, the sort that you see pictures of Russians wearing in the winter. But where would I wear one? We look at the produce market. Seeing the trays of summer berries I'm reminded of the open-air market that we saw in Bergen, Norway. However, the market here in Helsinki does not sell fish whereas the market in Bergen sells summer berries and fish.

As we sail out of Helsinki harbour in the evening we pass lots of very small rock islands that are barely visible and I'm glad we have the pilot on board.

Sailing into St Petersburg the following morning my first impressions are of run-down apartment buildings and ancient dock cranes of the type that I remember on the Auckland waterfront in the 1950s. Everything around the port looks more run-down than in Warnemünde and Gdansk. The docked ships that we pass are rusty and some look barely seaworthy. In fact the stern of one ship tied up at a pier is under the water.

The day is overcast with a brisk wind and the welcome from the Russian authorities matches the weather - decidedly chilly. But I'm getting slightly ahead of myself. As we walk down the gangway the St Petersburg Port Brass Band is on the wharf playing rousing American tunes like *When the saints go marching in.* It's great and we give them a hearty round of applause.

However, we step inside the customs shed and the warm welcome has gone, replaced by the frosty faces of the Russian customs officials. We have been warned that the customs officials are not friendly. Unless we have Russian visas (we haven't) we are only permitted to go ashore on organized tours. We aren't allowed to go ashore unaccompanied. Our passports are stamped and a red laminated card is placed inside saying something like 'Cruise passenger, temporary entry visa.' On our return to the ship the red card is removed and an outward stamp is placed beside the inwards one. Each day the process is repeated as we leave and return to the ship, although for some reason our passports are only stamped on the first day so it looks as though we have only spent one day in Russia instead of three.

I don't know why they don't allow cruise ship passengers to travel freely within the city. I heard several people say that they would have liked to go out for a walk, shopping or to a café. Similarly crew members who have days off while we are in St Petersburg are not allowed ashore. Surely every rouble spent by tourists helps the economy. It's not as though anyone from the ship would want to overstay and remain in the country. Illegal immigration may be a problem in many western countries but I can't see it being an attractive option in Russia.

Once we are in the bus we drive through the city streets. My first impression of central St Petersburg is that it is clean and well maintained. We see ongoing restoration of churches and modern shop windows in Nevsky Prospect. However, as we get further out of central St Petersburg things start to look a little worse for wear. There is an eclectic mix of cars on the street. Shiny new European and Japanese cars and beaten up, un-repaired old Ladas and Nivas. We pass several broken-down cars left on the side of the road. There are lots of old Soviet era trucks, but our tour bus is of a similar standard to the buses in other countries we visited.

We pass huge housing estates adjacent to industrial areas. The big multi-storeyed apartment blocks look depressing, but in reality they are probably no worse than the housing estates in the large English cities. I see the date 1977 on the side of one apartment block so I guess they were built in Soviet times.

One day as we are driving along, one of our guides mentions that for some people life today is not easier. In Soviet times people lived in free apartments, albeit often in cramped shared conditions. Now they need to pay rent or buy their apartment. Most people rent because if they buy a place and the outside of the building is not maintained their investment is at risk. Also older people are not able to get mortgages. There is a small pension for the elderly which may cover rent but not living expenses, forcing them to live with family members or work when they may otherwise be retired.

On our first day in St Petersburg we visit Catherine's Palace in Pushkin which is about one hour's drive from the city. Pushkin was occupied by the Germans in the Siege of Leningrad during World War II. Most of the art works were taken down by the Russians and safely stored before the palace was almost totally destroyed by the Germans. Today 29 of the 57 palace halls destroyed during the war have been restored.

The Palace was opened as a museum in 1918. I'm quite surprised that after murdering the Tsar and his family the communists did not also destroy all evidence of their existence. Similarly a large number of magnificent Russian Orthodox churches remain and yet the Soviet Union was officially an atheistic state. One of our guides tells us that because of the teaching at school, which she referred to as brainwashing, she is an atheist. Yet it appears that the churches functioned openly and were tolerated by the regime. Today churches are being restored to their former glory and many Russians actively worship in the Russian Orthodox church.

Catherine's Palace was the summer residence of the Tsars. The palace was expanded and renovated by Peter the Great's daughter the Empress Elizabeth and then expanded and further renovated by Catherine. We arrive at the palace and walk briskly to the entrance. We have a scheduled entry time for our tour and our guide is anxious that we don't miss it.

There are bus loads of tourists waiting to enter the palace. The queuing is not as orderly as at Buckingham Palace. Once inside the palace we all need to put covers (they are operating theatre overshoes) over our shoes to protect the surface of the floors. There are lots of people in a small room all trying to put the covers over their shoes. I need to sit down to do this otherwise I'll fall over. Luckily there is a wooden bench and as soon as someone stands up I quickly take my place on the bench and struggle to reach down and put the covers over my shoes and quickly move off to join our group.

We are given whisper kits (earphones and a small receiver) so that we can hear what our guide is saying. The overshoes are slippery and as we climb the marble staircase I'm too busy hauling myself up the stairs and trying not to slip over to really appreciate the beauty of the staircase. The palace rooms are truly magnificent. There are rooms with gilt embossing on the walls, huge mirrors, carved wood and plaster features. In many of the rooms there are blue and white tiled Dutch stoves, however we are told that these are just fashionable ornaments and were not used to heat this summer palace.

The amber room is probably the most well known room in Catherine's Palace, and it was used as a study. The walls were constructed of perfectly fitted pieces of amber. During World War II the Germans occupied Pushkin and it is said that they dismantled the amber panels and shipped them to Germany. The Amber room has been completely re-built and was re-opened to the public in 2003. We are not allowed to take photos in this room and we pass through it fairly quickly. My impressions are that it was dark and a little claustrophobic, although this may be due to the numbers of people who were in the room as photos show it in a different light.

Many people in our group make comments about the extravagance of the palaces, linking it with the revolution. Having recently read a couple of novels set in the misery of pre-revolutionary rural Russia I can understand the plight of the ordinary people, although in no way do I condone the murder of the Tsar and his family or what has subsequently happened over the years in the Soviet Union.

On our way out of the Palace Mum and I stand in line for the ladies' toilets for about ten minutes wondering if the group will leave without us. As we are waiting other tour guides come in calling for members of their party and we eventually get back to our meeting place with minutes to spare. Later I hear that a lady had her wallet taken from her handbag by pick pockets while she was waiting in line to use the toilet.

On our second day in Russia Mum is up early to go on a day trip to Moscow. I choose not to go because it's a 16 hour round trip and includes a Russian dinner with vodka in the evening before the return flight to St Petersburg. I know that I won't be able to eat the meal or drink the vodka and after 16 hours I will be exhausted. Mum goes off on the trip to Moscow and I have a leisurely breakfast in the Grand Dining Room followed by a quiet morning on the ship. While I am in our cabin getting ready for my afternoon tour to the cathedrals the door opens and Mum comes in looking absolutely shattered.

"We didn't go" she says. After a three hour wait at St Petersburg airport for a plane that didn't come, 17 of the 68 people in the party cancelled and returned to the ship. The others in the group eventually make it to Moscow on another plane and they get back to the ship at 1am. It appears that the lost plane was the Pulkovo Airlines Tupolev Tu-154 that crashed in Ukraine a few days earlier and no one had replaced it!!! Also several people had been killed by a bomb in a Moscow market place a few days earlier too so I'm glad Mum didn't go. Mum rests in our cabin while I go on the afternoon tour to the cathedrals.

First we visit St. Isaac's Cathedral. This is the fourth largest cathedral in the world after St Peter's in Rome, St Paul's in London and Santa María de las Flores in Florence, all of which I have visited over the years. St. Isaac's Cathedral will accommodate 14,000 standing worshippers. It was closed in the 1930s and is now open as a museum. Inside there are amazing incredibly detailed mosaic icons, 19th century paintings and columns made of malachite and lapis lazuli. Inside the main altar is a stunning stained glass window of the Resurrected Christ.

Back in the bus we go around the corner to the Kazan Cathedral located on Nevsky Prospect, the main thoroughfare of St Petersburg. The cathedral was named after the mother and child icon called Kazan Mother of God. The men in our group are asked to take their hats off as we enter and several ladies in the group cover their heads. Inside the Cathedral Russian women, heads covered with scarves, kiss icons and light candles. A priest stands beside the Kazan Mother of God icon. A long line of mainly female worshippers inch their way forward to kiss the icon and have a few words with the priest. Our guide tells us that unlike Catholic priests, Russian Orthodox priests must be married.

I wander around looking at the icons and wonder how this compares with the Greek Orthodox church next door to where I live in Sydney. I don't think that the Greek women cover their heads in church. Our guide shows us the icon of Tsar Nicholas II and the Romanov family. She tells us that in 2000 the Bishops of the Russian Orthodox Church recognized Tsar Nicholas, Empress Alexandra and their five children as saints. She mentions that this is a controversial decision as some people say it is too soon after their death to make them saints. Also there are still Russians alive who knew them. Others believe that Nicholas' reign was weak and prone to extravagance and indifference to the plight of Russia's needy and that these things ultimately led to the revolution and their execution. Regardless of the rights and wrongs of their sainthood, I wonder if perhaps it is Russia's way of saying "sorry" to them. A few days later in a church in Tallinn I see another icon of the Romanov family and find it a moving experience to look at them and remember their fate.

The third cathedral we visit is the Church of the Resurrection of Jesus Christ, commonly known as The Church of Our Saviour of the Spilled Blood. It is a typically Russian cathedral with nine beautiful gold and enamel mosaic onion-dome cupolas, whereas the other two cathedrals look more like St Peter's in Rome or St Paul's in London. The cathedral sits on the site where Tsar Alexander II was murdered on the 1st of March, 1881. The Tsar was mortally wounded by a bomb thrown by the terrorists from the People's Will revolutionist organization. We see the preserved fragments of railings and the cobblestone pavement where the Emperor fell. The cathedral was damaged and closed soon after the revolution of 1917 and was used as a storehouse for many years. Restoration began in 1970 and was completed in 1991.

Later that afternoon, back on the ship, I need to re-charge the battery on my digital camera but I don't have the right power plug for the ship's American power points. I go to the reception desk on deck 4 with a note. *I've lost my voice. Do you have an adaptor for my plug that I can borrow? I would try to buy one at the shop but it won't be open till we leave St Petersburg*. They don't have an adaptor but the receptionist arranges for the ship's electrician to charge up my battery. As I'm leaving a crew member passes saying that the dome of a church is on fire. He goes out on to deck four to look. I follow him out but don't see anything as we are too low. I go up to deck 10 and from here I can see the whole dome of a church totally engulfed by flames. The flames are leaping up metres above the dome into the sky. The fire is over the other side of the river from where the three cathedrals that I visited are. Someone mentions that it is a church that is being restored, and they wonder if the fire was caused by a spark from a welder's torch.

On our third day in Russia we visit Peter the Great's Palace at Peterhof. Peterhof is outside St Petersburg overlooking the Gulf of Finland. Like Catherine's Palace, Peterhof was damaged during WWII and its interiors have been meticulously restored to their breathtaking former glory. Fortunately the treasures of both Peterhof and Catherine's Palace were stored in the basement of the Hermitage and St Isaac's Cathedral before the Germans laid siege to the city.

On the way out to the palace our guide talks to us about the siege of Leningrad which lasted for a total of 900 days, from September 8 1941 until January 27 1944. She tells us that of a population of three million people at least 600,000 people died of cold and starvation. In just two months of the winter in 1942, 200,000 people died in Leningrad of cold and starvation yet despite all of the terrible hardships, the city's war industries still continued to work and the city did not surrender. There must be many older people still alive in St Petersburg who lived through those dreadful times.

It's a sunny Saturday afternoon when we visit Peterhof. The palace is set in a wonderful park with fountains, statues and pavilions running down to the Baltic seashore. The fountains are spectacular and have been compared to those at Versailles. There are lots of St Petersburg locals here enjoying a sunny afternoon in the gardens too.

We line up and await our turn to enter the Palace. It doesn't seem to be as crowded as Catherine's Palace was the other day. We put on our overshoes again and plug in our whisper sets. The interior of the palace is every bit as spectacular as Catherine's Palace but it's the gardens that stick in my mind. Everything has been so painstakingly restored to its former glory.

Despite my criticism of the unfriendliness of the Russian customs officials and their restrictive entry visas I am impressed with the restoration of these treasures. It is laudable that a Soviet regime that could have easily gone the way of the Taliban and destroyed all trace of cultural treasures that, in their opinion, represented an undesirable element of the past, has supported such painstaking restoration and preservation of the past.

As we drive back to St Petersburg through dormitory suburbs of depressing high rise apartment buildings and adjacent industrial areas I overhear some of the Americans in our group saying how lucky they are not to have been born somewhere like this.

While in St Petersburg I was determined that I would not 'overdo it' by trying to do and see too much. The choice of tours that I went on was influenced mainly by the time of day and the duration of the tour. In particular, I missed going to the Hermitage. I missed an evening at the Russian Ballet, *Swan Lake*. I missed a Champagne reception and musical evening at Catherine's Palace followed by dinner at a local restaurant, I also missed an evening of Russian song and dance and of course as mentioned earlier, I didn't go to Moscow.

As we sail out of St Petersburg past the same sad looking ships and old cranes I think *there have been lots of changes since perestroika but there is still a long way to go.* The locals don't seem to have a sense of humour. Several people have mentioned that they haven't seen anyone smiling. I'm not surprised though, life still seems to be hard. It will probably take another generation or two for real changes to be seen.

On Sunday morning we sail in to Tallinn, Estonia. After Russia this is like a breath of fresh air. We walk off the ship, no passport inspection, we can just go. I think *what a wonderful opportunity St Petersburg could have to open its doors to the Western world, allowing tourists to come and go freely like this. There is such a wealth of cultural treasure in St Petersburg to be shared with the world.*

We meet our Estonian guide and travel in the bus to the Old Town at the top of the hill. Our guide seems to have a wonderful sense of humour and as she talks I get the impression that she has put the past behind her and with no bitterness she is just getting on with things, whereas I got the impression that the Russians are still looking over their shoulder, not completely trusting President Putin (because of his KGB past) and the new regime.

Our guide tells us that Estonia has had freedom from the Soviets for 15 years. In Soviet times people often waited up to 20 years just to get a telephone in their house. Now almost everyone has a Nokia cell phone. She explains how Estonian people are related to Hungarians and Finns and they are not at all like Russians. She says that the Estonians and Finns came from Hungary, the Estonians stopped when they reached the water and the Finns are those who could swim!

Our walking tour of Tallinn and the Old Town starts at the top of the hill. We look down at the medieval city walls, the watch towers, spires and cobblestoned streets. It's Sunday and we hear the church bells ringing for the morning service. Even though the service is in progress we are able to go inside the Russian Orthodox church. The church is filled with the magnificent singing of the choir. There are no seats, the worshippers are standing and wandering around. Ladies with scarves over their heads pass by icons, crossing themselves, lighting candles, kissing the icon and murmuring prayers, seemingly oblivious to the influx of foreign tourists. I watch with interest. Living next door to the Greek Orthodox church in Kogarah I have noticed how people appear to wander in and out during the Sunday service which seems to last from 8am until 11am.

I look for and, as mentioned earlier, find the icon of the Romanov family. Tsar Nicholas II, Alexandra, and all their five children are considered to be martyrs in the Russian Orthodox Church for their devotion and exemplary Christian lifestyle. They are dressed in long white gowns and have halos around their heads. Having recently read a book about the search for Anastasia, the Tsar's daughter whom it was thought may have survived the massacre, I find it a rather poignant reminder of the tragedy.

Out of the church we look at the castle on the other side of the square. The castle is now the seat of Estonia's parliament. Mum asks the guide if we can go inside for a look but it's Sunday and it's closed. Our guide leads us down the hill to the Lower Town through narrow cobbled alleys inside the town wall. Every hundred yards or so a fold up wooden seat is attached to the wall, a modern addition for people walking up hill.

We emerge in the town square which is dominated by the 15th century town hall. The street cafes lining the square are crowded with locals and tourists enjoying the sunny Sunday morning. I'm only sorry that I can't join them and have coffee or a beer in the sun. We meet up with our guide again and walk to the bus for our trip back to the ship. In the afternoon Mum goes out for a walk (unlike Russia, here she can just walk off the ship) and I sit in the Horizons lounge enjoying the view.

Overnight we sail to Stockholm, our final port. In the morning, the sail into Stockholm is spectacular. For several hours we pass through the archipelago of islands. There are about 24,000 islands surrounding Stockholm. Many of the islands are uninhabited, on others there are holiday houses. The houses get larger as we get closer to Stockholm and I wonder if people live in them permanently and commute in to Stockholm.

Having previously been to Stockholm Mum and I don't book to go on any of the ship's tours, as we can find our own way around. We get the local bus into the city and go to the Tourist information centre where we buy two-day Stockholm cards. These cards give us 48 hours use of buses, trains, some ferries and entry to many of Stockholm's must-see attractions. As it is raining we catch the bus back to the ship and enjoy a leisurely final day on the ship.

That evening we pack our suitcases and put them out for collection. We can only carry hand luggage off the ship. We are up early the following morning and after breakfast we wait in the *Regatta* lounge for the bus to our hotel to be called.

A whole bus load of us arrive at the Hilton Hotel Slussen. *Go and check in, I'll look after the bags* I tell Mum. Amazingly Mum is at the head of the queue and we are checked in quickly. The bags are another story. We decide to go up to our room and come back later for them.

A bit later I go down to arrange for our bags to be brought up to our room and I also check our airport pick up times with the Oceania tours representative. He has a pick up time of 15:45 for both Mum and me. I inform him that Mum's flight departs at 14:30 and he makes a phone call to arrange a separate pick up for her at 11:30.

Tuesday is a lovely sunny day and Mum and I travel by public bus from Slussen to Skansen. We wait no more than three or four minutes before a bus comes along. At Kungstradgardsg we get off the bus and in less than one minute bus 47 comes along and we are on our way to Skansen. In a note to Mum I say *See how easy it was for us to change buses? You can't do that in Auckland.* In the evening we are having dinner at the hotel. Our table overlooks the bridge connecting the Slussen area with Gamla Stan and I point to the trains crossing the bridge and say to Mum *there is a train every 2 minutes.* We talk about how good the public transport is in Stockholm. *You need to start talking to local politicians about getting cheap frequent public transport for Auckland,* I suggest to Mum. *When Dylan worked at Bayswater the Birkenhead bus arrived in Takapuna 5 minutes after the Bayswater bus had gone. It's hopeless!* I tell her.

Skansen is an open air museum. Mum and I visited it when we were in Stockholm in 2001, however we didn't see everything and Mum is keen to return. With our Stockholm card we have free entry. Skansen is located on the side of a hill and I find it quite difficult walking up the slight incline of cobbled paths. Aided by my walking stick I struggle to keep up with Mum. I don't let on to her that I'm struggling; it's hard to admit that your almost 80 year old mother is fitter than you are.

I'm interested in seeing the houses, farmsteads and the replica of a Swedish mid-19th century town, whereas Mum wants to see the Scandinavian animals. First we visit Town Quarters. There are workshops and dwellings side by side. We watch cabinet makers and glass-blowers in their traditional workshops demonstrating their skills. I'm interested in the pharmacy where a girl dressed in a traditional costume explains how the pharmacist and his apprentice made medicines from local plants. A pharmacist was available 24 hours a day and she shows us the small bed where the pharmacist on duty slept overnight. At the bakery Mum buys a bun and a couple of traditional biscuits for lunch and we sit on a bench in the sun, Mum eating her lunch and me having a can of Jevity.

Then we follow the signs to the Scandinavian animals. We smell the animals before we see them. In an enclosure are several huge bison and lots of pigs. There are wolves in the next enclosure and we see a couple lying on the ground amongst the bushes. They look like German Shepherd dogs. There are also some wolverines in their own enclosure. I find the animals are a bit disappointing and I'm keen to move on.

We look at the various farm houses that have been shipped piece by piece to the museum and re-assembled. Many of the houses only have one room. Some are two family duplexes, with two rooms separated by an entry lobby. It's hard to imagine whole families living in one room, particularly during the long winters. We also see Skogaholm Manor, from central Sweden, which consists of a main building, two wings, two pavilions and a summerhouse. It has a French garden, a kitchen garden and a small English park. Nearby is the Älvros Farmstead from northern Sweden. There are several buildings: a farmhouse, stable, cow shed, hay barn and storage rooms, grouped to form a square, enclosed courtyard.

Skansen is a place that you can come back to again and again, there is always something of interest. We have had a lovely day. Outside we see the number 47 bus waiting at the terminus. (Skansen is the end of the route). We hop on the bus showing the driver our Stockholm cards. He says something in Swedish that we don't understand, but it seems as though he is trying to tell us that we can't get on the bus. Mum speaks to him but clearly he is one of the very few Swedish people who don't speak English. Eventually he indicates that we can stay on the bus. Some other people come along to get on the bus and whatever he says to them, they get off the bus and walk along the road. We stay on the bus. Shortly the bus moves off and stops at a bus stop just along the road and the other people get on. He must have been telling us that we had to get on at the bus stop I tell Mum. Never mind, we are on the right bus and we retrace our route back to the hotel.

It's such a lovely day and I suggest to Mum that we sit in the sun. We cross the road to the waterfront and sit on a bench in the sun watching the ferry boats come and go. Stockholm is such a beautiful city.

This has been a truly wonderful cruise. My favourite places have been London and Stockholm both of which I've visited before and Tallin, Estonia. I loved the attitude of the Estonian people and I am impressed with how they have progressed during their 15 years of freedom compared with Russia. I am also impressed with the attitude of our Estonian guide, who seemed to have no bitterness towards the past and was just keen to get on with things, whereas it appears that the Russians are still distrustful of Putin and afraid to step out of line. We didn't see any smiling faces in Russia. I found Russia distinctly unfriendly towards tourists. Warnemünde, in former East Germany, and Gdansk still show traces of their former Soviet connections but the people seem to be happier than the Russians.

On the day of our departure I'm not happy that they have allowed enough time for me to get to the airport. I don't want to have to rush and I'd rather be there early. I write a note for Alonzo the Oceania representative. I really would like to go to the airport earlier than 15:45. I'm happy to go with someone who is leaving earlier. An elderly Chinese couple from Perth are leaving for the airport at 12:30. That's too early. I write. He phones the limo company but they are unable to pick me up after 12:30 and before 15:45 and I decide to go with the Chinese couple. Maybe I can get an earlier flight to Heathrow I think. If not I can sit in the British Airways Lounge and use the computer.

On arrival at the airport I hand the guy at the check in counter an note saying: I know I'm early and I'm happy to go on an earlier flight. In Australia this often works especially if you are booked on a peak hour flight and want to swap for an off peak flight. "The type of ticket that you have can't be changed" he says. *Never mind.* I think. *I'll use the computer in the British Airways Lounge.*

Going through the security x-ray they put my backpack through the x-ray three times. I have three cans of Jevity and a bottle of water in my backpack and I'm expecting to be questioned about one or other. However, after the third time the man passes my backpack to me saying "OK." Once through security the only lounge is Finnair. However, Finnair is a One World partner airline so that's OK. When compared to the Qantas Club lounges the Finnair lounge is stark. There are no floor coverings. *This wooden floor must be cold in winter* I think. The furnishings are pretty stark too but there are three computers. I hurry over and sit down at a computer. After paying 95 US cents per minute to send email on the ship, free internet access is great.

Logging on to the internet I'm surprised to see that the words on the screen are in another language. I guess it's Swedish or Finnish but I wouldn't know the difference. However, the fields are the same and pretty soon I'm logged on to my hotmail and replying to emails that I put off doing while on the ship because of the cost. With personal emails out of the way I log on to my work emails. New emails total 222! I systematically go through deleting all the junk emails and scanning the rest for anything urgent. That done I sit down and read until it's time to board the plane.

To reach the departure gate I need to pass through passport control. The man flicks through the pages in my passport several times and then says "I can see in and out of Poland but I can't see a stamp for entering Sweden." Unsure what he is getting at I point to the Russian stamps which are the most recent stamps in my passport. "I don't care about Russia" he says and just stamps my passport. Surely he knows how passports aren't always needed when passing from one EU country to another. On the whole cruise the only places where our passports were stamped were entering and leaving Britain, entering Belgium, entering and leaving Poland and entering and leaving Russia on the first day only. In all the other countries we could just leave the ship without passing through any border control.

I had hoped to eat dinner on the 6:30 British Airways flight to Heathrow. However, the meal served is a boxed ham and cheese roll. I don't even try to eat one. I ask for a can of coke and I am given a 150ml can of coke. There are no earphones and no movie on this two hour flight. Luckily I have my own earphones with me and when I plug them in the audio system is working. Compared to British Airways, Qantas easily wins. Even on a one hour dinner time Qantas flight between Melbourne and Sydney a hot meal is served (not that I eat it), the cans of coke are 375 ml., there are complimentary earphones and the TV news is shown. I've flown within Europe before and even business class wasn't as good as Qantas or Air New Zealand.

I am asked, presumably at random, to fill in a British Airways customer satisfaction questionnaire. The questions don't exactly address the issues that are of concern to me, however, I indicate that the meal service is not up to my expectation.

Arriving at Heathrow's Terminal 1 I walk for what seems like miles to the transfer desk. Here I need to pass through the security x-ray screening. There is a list indicating the items that, under the tightened security measures, are not permitted. The list includes bottled water. There are abandoned water bottles lying on the floor and everyone is taking their shoes off. By the time it is my turn to pass through the screening I have not had time to remove my water bottle. I remove my shoes thinking *They will search my bag anyway when they see the tins.* I put my backpack, shoes and walking stick on the moving x-ray belt and hobble through the metal scanner. My bag passes straight through the x-ray and I pick it up and go.

In the transfer bus to Terminal 4 it seems as though we have driven halfway across London before we finally reach the terminal. More miles of corridors to be walked along at Terminal 4. I see two police officers, a man and a woman, in flak jackets, machine guns at the ready, patrolling the terminal. I also see a couple of Islamic women covered from head to toe in black gowns with only their eyes showing. I assume they are women but it's hard to tell. *Will they be subject to extra security?* I wonder. Despite the increased airline security following the arrests in London of people suspected of plotting to blow up transatlantic planes, I have had surprisingly trouble-free travel to and from Heathrow. I have had more hassles passing through airline security on Australian domestic flights and agricultural inspections at Auckland International Airport. I change my Euros and US dollars to Australian dollars, spend loose change on some sweets – the British make good lollies – and I only have time to go to the toilet and it's time to board QF 2 to Sydney via Bangkok.

I'm back in my 18A seat in the back row of the upper deck and I have an empty seat beside me. I eat dinner, put my seat back in the fully reclined position and sleep well until we are approaching Bangkok. The captain tells us there is a mid-afternoon storm and we have to circle for a while. Below I see green fields. From the plane window I see flashes of lightning in the distance. Knowing how Sydney airport sometimes closes during electrical storms I have visions of being diverted to somewhere like Ho Chi Minh City, however we do land in Bangkok. In the Qantas Club I log on to a computer and send some more emails.

There is an email from Kevin saying that he went with Dylan to Starship Hospital last night to see Aaliyah who yesterday had

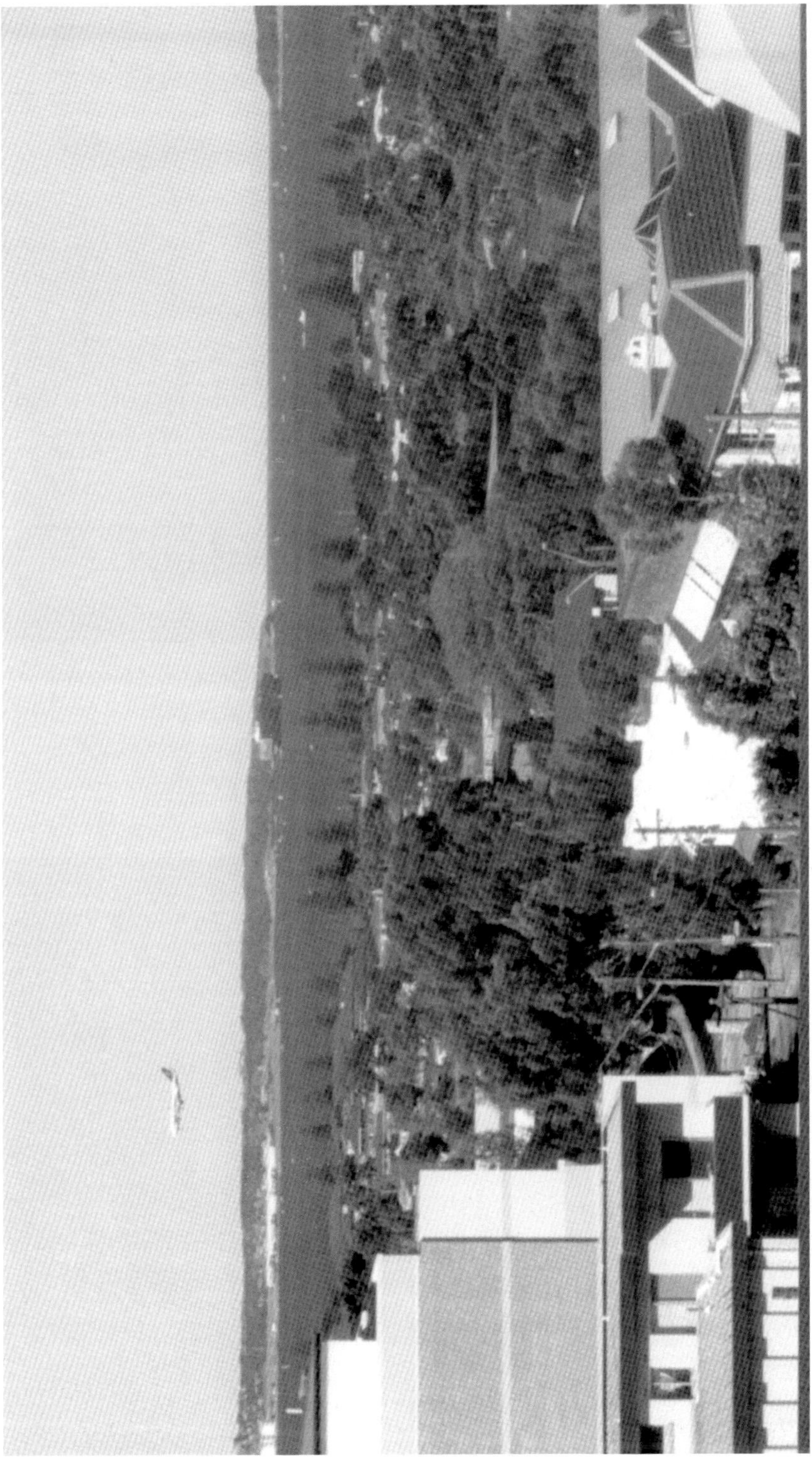

Above: *The wonderful view from my sixth floor apartment of Sydney's Botany Bay. A container ship is heading out to sea and a plane is coming in from the south to land at Sydney International Airport. The Norfolk pines in the middle of the picture line the seaward side of The Grand Parade at Brighton-le-Sands Beach.*

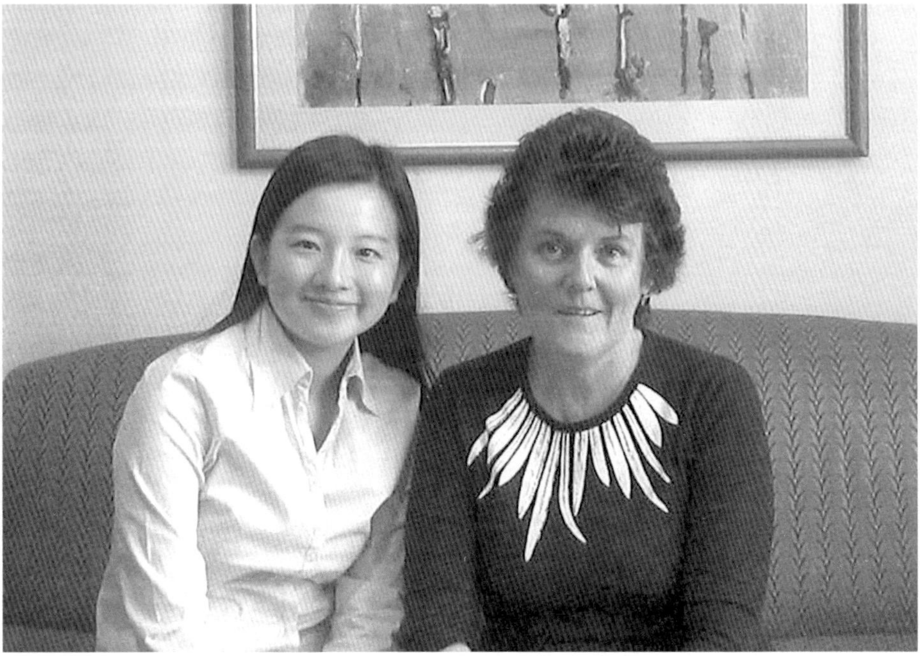

Above: *I spent a week in Melbourne training Judy and every time I tried to speak to her, I coughed.*

Below: *The Greek Fair. My apartment building is next to the Greek Church in Belgrave Street, Kogarah. My balcony (arrow) overlooks the roof of the church to a wonderful view.*

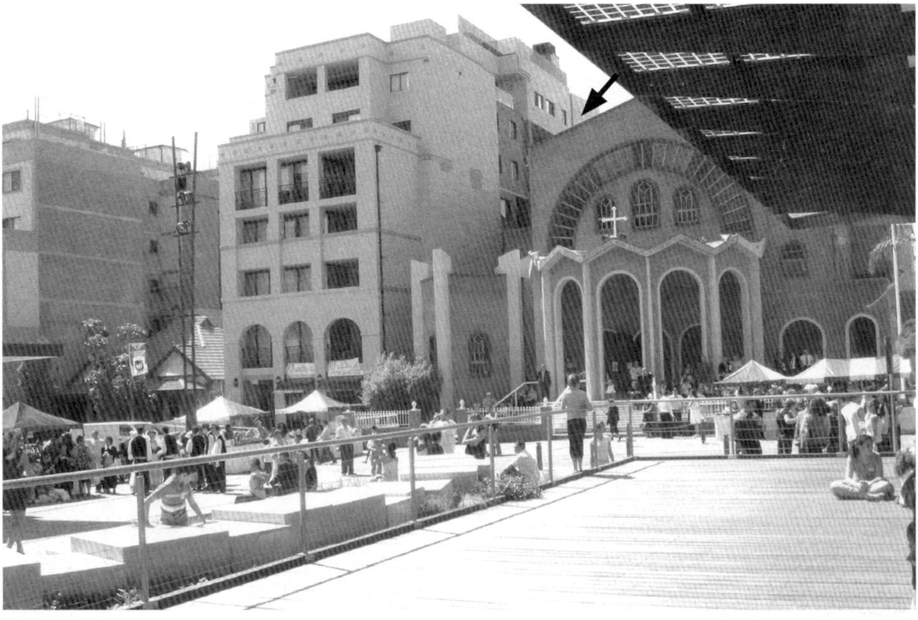

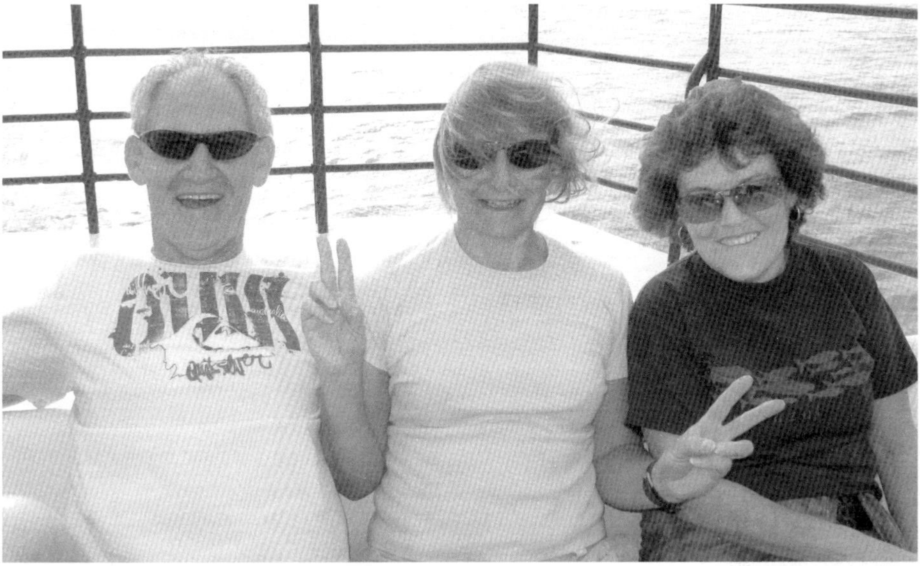

Above: *With Jenni and Francis on our snorkelling trip to the outer Great Barrier Reef.*

Below: *Kevin and I arriving at Hiva Oa, Marquesas Islands, French Polynesia; January 2006.*

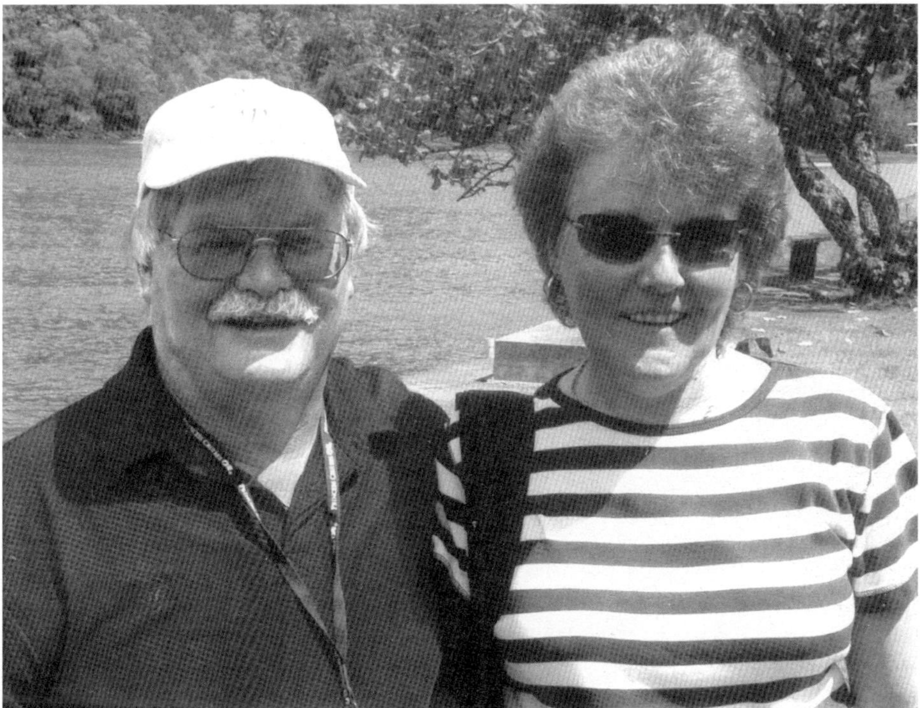

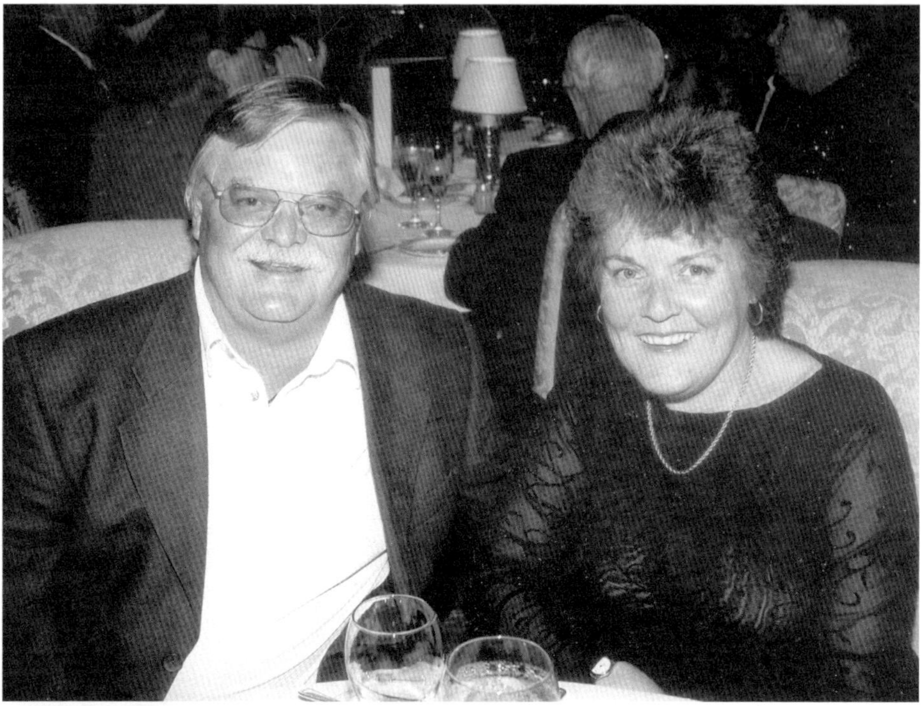

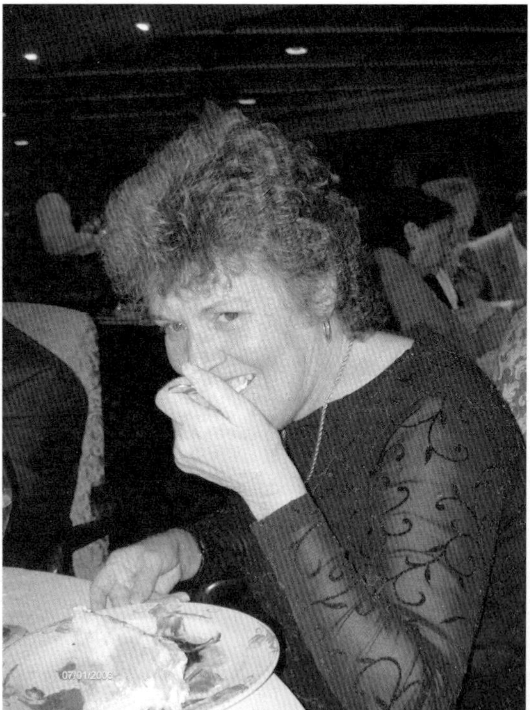

Above: *Kevin and I at the Farewell Dinner on Tahitian Princess; January 2006*

Left: *Here I am tucking in to a second helping of Baked Alaska at the Farewell Dinner on Tahitian Princess; January 2006.*

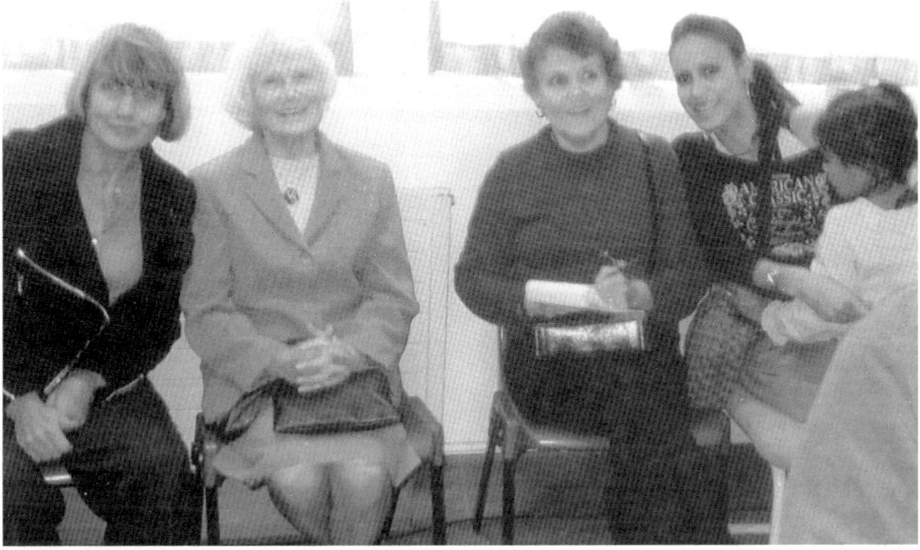

Above: *Four generations; Mum with Jenni on the left, me on the right with my notebook and pen. Emma is next to me with Aaliyah sitting on her knee*

Below: *Making friends with a koala at Featherdale Wildlife Park, Sydney; October 2006.*

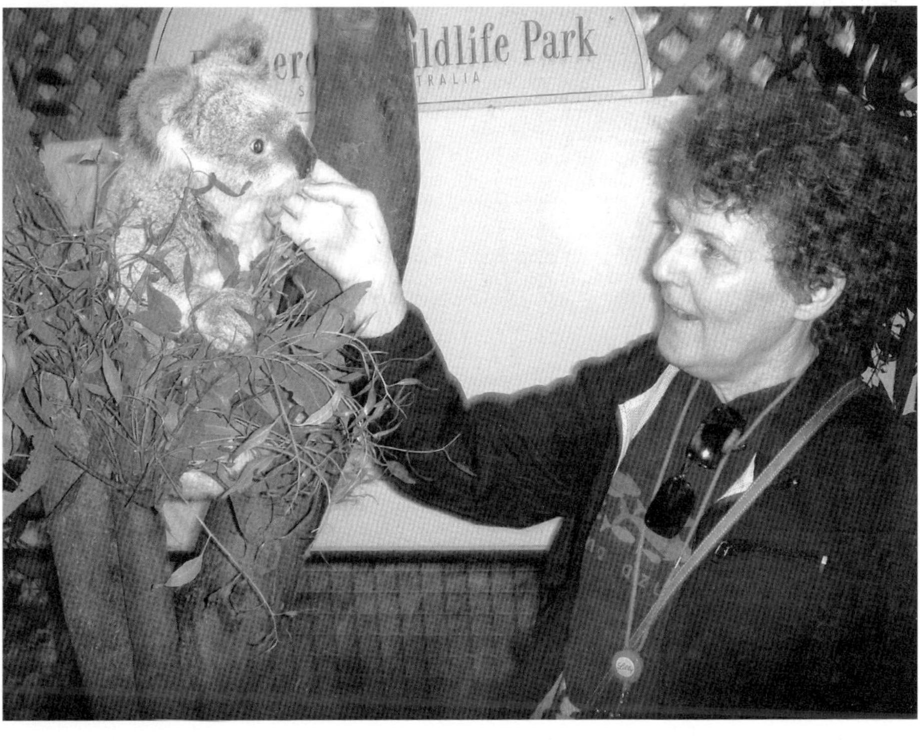

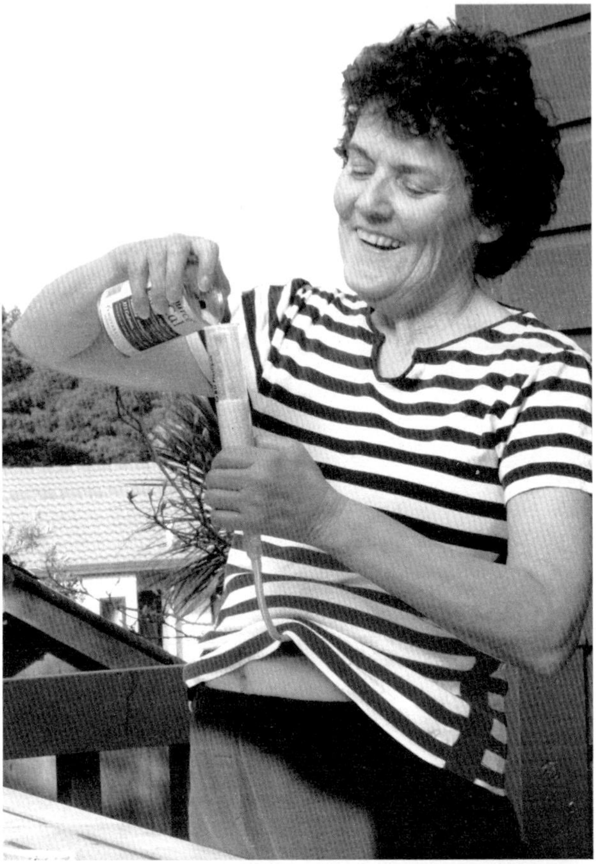

Right: *Feeding with a 'PEG' becomes part of my daily routine.*

Below: *36 cans of Jevity for my trip packed in a photocopy box. I've stuck a label off a can and a typed note with my name and destination etc on the top of the box. The letter from the dietician verifying the contents is taped to the side of the box.*

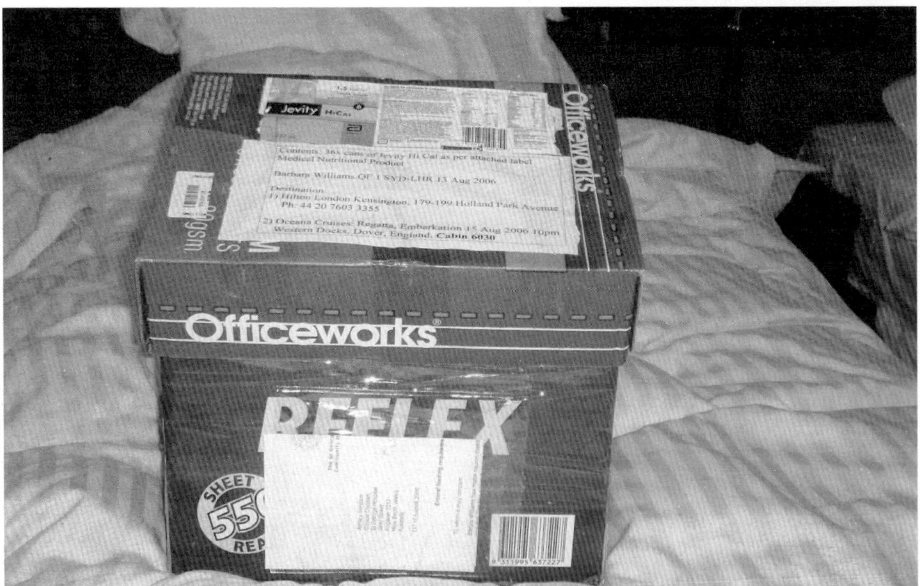
Jevity HiCal
Officeworks
Contents: 36x cans of Jevity Hi Cal as per attached label
Medical Nutritional Product
Barbara Williams QF 1 SYD-LHR 13 Aug 2006
Destination
1) Hilton London Kensington, 179-199 Holland Park Avenue
Ph: 44 20 7603 3355
2) Oceana Cruises: Regatta, Embarkation 15 Aug 2006 10pm
Western Docks, Dover, England. Cabin 6030
Officeworks
REFLEX

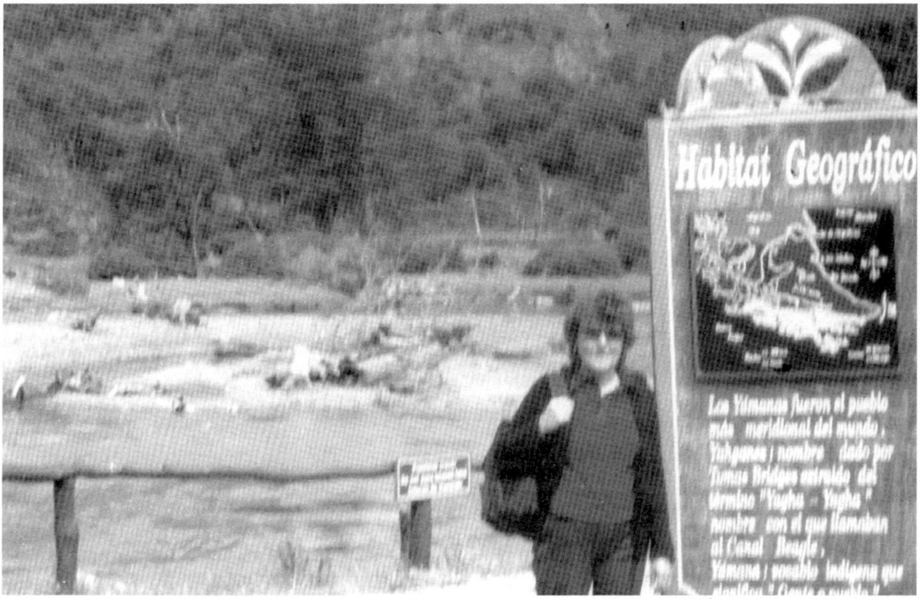

Above: *At a national park, Tierra del Fuego, during the South American cruise; January 2005.*

Below: *Mum and I in Tallinn, Estonia; August 2006.*

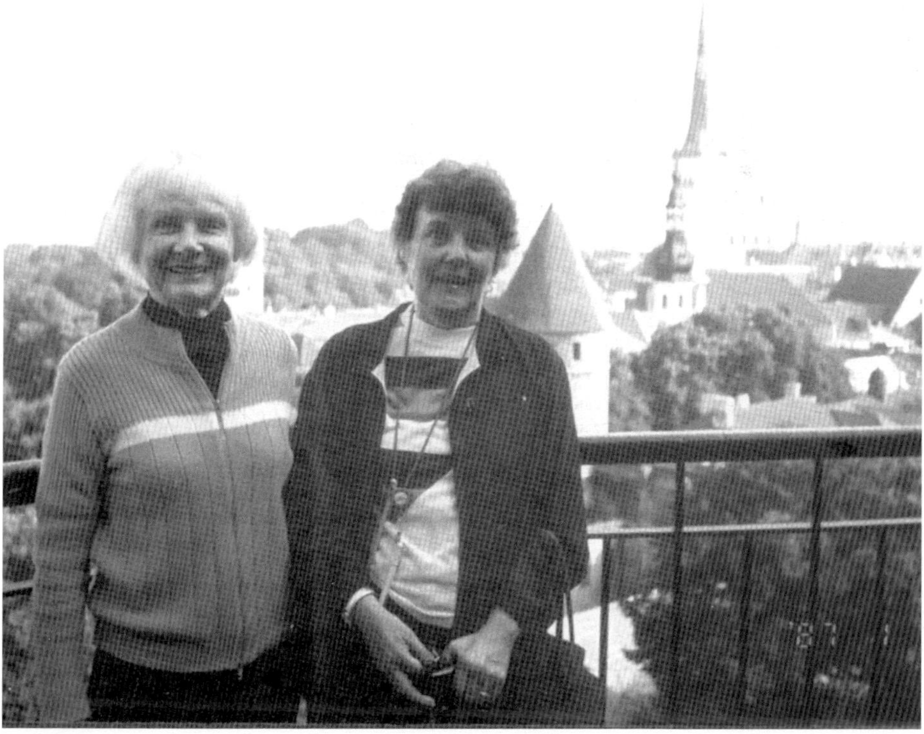

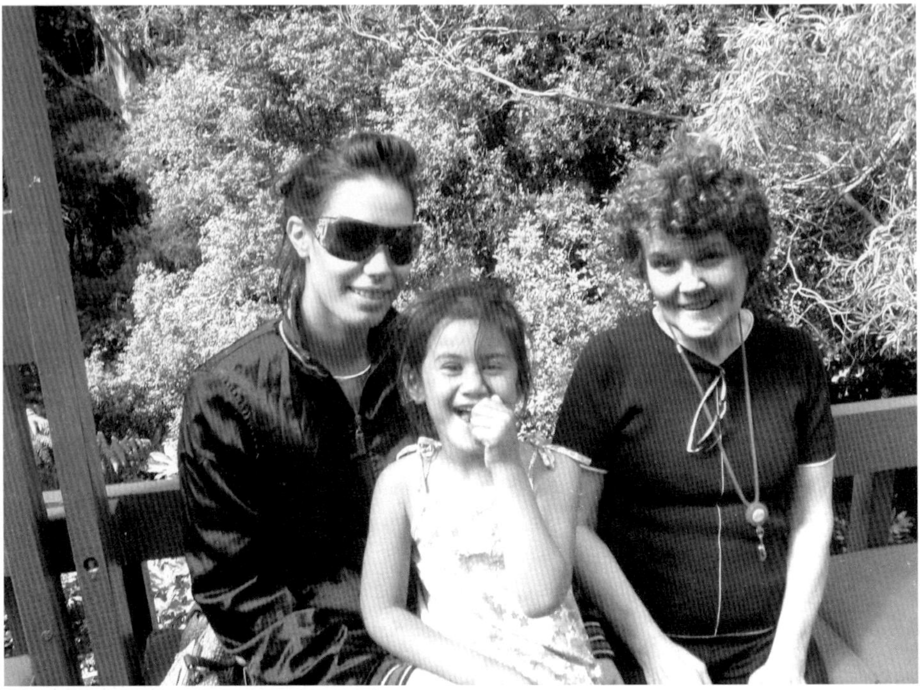

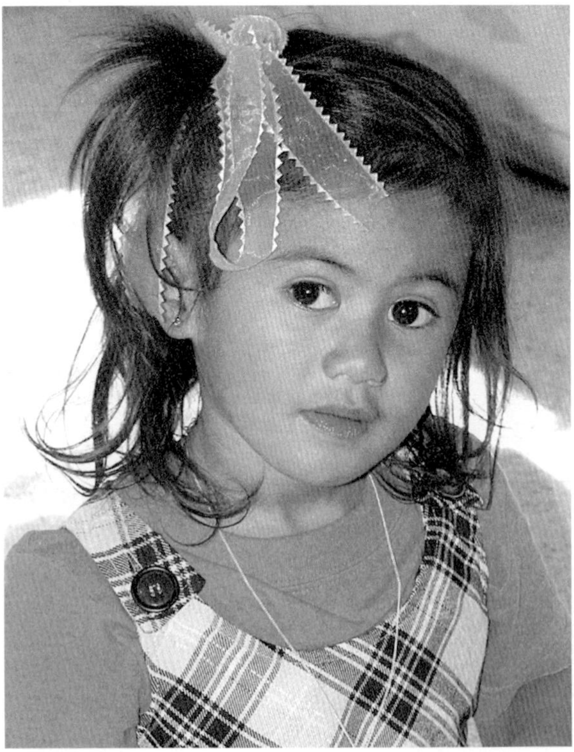

Above: *With Emma and Aaliyah celebrating my 55th birthday; December 2006.*

Left: *Aaliyah on her third birthday.*

broken her elbow at Kindy. He said that the surgeon could not believe Aaliyah was only four years old because she is so articulate and big for her age - he thought she was about seven. Then when Emma was arranging to stay at the Starship he questioned her age and said "You have to be over 16 to stay with a child." He thought that Emma who is 23 was Aaliyah's sister! Fortunately Aaliyah has treated the episode as a big adventure and goes home the next day.

Back on the plane I'm hoping for an empty seat beside me again but at the last minute a man comes along. He takes one look at the seat and says "I'm travelling with my friend. Would you like to swap seats with him?" I shake my head. Next the other man asks the man next to him if he will swap, this man also says no. They are a couple of middle aged 'Aussie blokes.' They stand in the aisle drinking Champagne and talking loudly. *I hope they don't carry on like this all night* I think to myself. Then the man next to me has a Bloody Mary for a pre-dinner drink followed by one or two glasses of red wine with dinner. I'm determined not to be intimidated by him and luckily he goes to sleep shortly after dinner and sleeps for the rest of the flight. I sleep well too.

In the morning we are due to land in Sydney at 6am. We start our descent and I return my seat to the upright position and put my shoes on. The captain's voice comes over the speaker "Sorry folks, we have been asked to hold for ten minutes. There is a lot of traffic around when the curfew comes off." Officially there are no landings at Sydney airport between 11pm and 6am. However, from my kitchen window I often see two or three planes coming in at about 5am when I'm taking my morning Riluzole. Anyway we go round in circles and in due course we come in from the south over Botany Bay to land.

While standing in the queue of people waiting to get off the plane there is an announcement "Would the following people please contact a Qantas representative at the gate" …a dozen or so names are read out and I feel sure my name will be in the list. Sure enough at the and of the list I hear "Williams" I know immediately what it is – my luggage is lost! I show the Qantas representative my *I've lost my voice* card and my British Airways boarding pass and I'm handed a card:

> **PLEASE GO TO QANTAS BAGGAGE SERVICES IN THE CUSTOMS HALL AFTER CLEARING IMMIGRATION FORMALITIES**

"They will be waiting for you," the lady says. Yes, they are waiting for me and about 20 others who are in the queue in front of me. Bloody Heathrow! In all the years that I've been travelling this is the third time my luggage has been lost and each time it has involved transfer from one flight to another at London's Heathrow airport.

The first time in the mid 1990's I was flying United Airlines from Chicago's O'Hare airport to Rome. Our departure from O'Hare was delayed for some reason and I missed my onward Lufthansa connection at Heathrow to Rome via Frankfurt. At O'Hare I had been upgraded from Business to First class and on arrival at Heathrow I was very swiftly transferred by car to a British airways flight going directly to Rome but my luggage didn't make it. Fortunately the luggage turned up in Rome in time for a change of clothes before the meeting.

The second time in 2000 I was en-route to Amsterdam via Heathrow and my luggage did not make the connection. I was spending the long Easter weekend with friends in Hattem, central Netherlands. For the whole Easter weekend I had to wear the clothes that I had travelled from New Zealand in. Fortunately my luggage was delivered on Easter Monday in time for me to travel by train to Brussels where I was attending a meeting.

The Sydney Qantas baggage services man who is dealing with me is very helpful. In the course of our conversation I write *Heathrow always loses bags in transit*. "Yes, it keeps us in a job" he replies and assures me that the bag will be delivered on Saturday between

4pm and 8pm. I guess this is a daily occurrence with flights from Heathrow.

With only my carry on back pack I try to join the queue of people for customs screening. I have never seen such chaos at Sydney airport. Everywhere there are people with luggage trolleys piled high milling around trying to reach the customs queue. It's just gridlock! It takes me two hours to clear immigration, customs and the taxi line. Finally, I'm home. It's Friday morning, I log on to my computer and start work.

On Saturday morning I get a phone call "Hello Mrs. Williams it's John here from Qantas. I was dealing with your lost bag yesterday. I have your bag right here. It has your Qantas Club name tag on it. The courier will deliver it between 4pm and 7pm today. He will text you the exact time of his arrival." Sure enough at 4:30 in the afternoon I get a text message **"courier: b there half hr or less"** Just before 5pm I wander down to the front door thinking that it will be easier if I'm waiting there when the courier arrives. As I'm walking along the corridor to the front door I see the courier approaching the door pulling my suitcase behind him!

Back in my apartment I see that my suitcase has a British Airways tag on it

TRANSER AT LHR TO

TERMINAL 4

SHORT.

Yet, clearly my bag did not reach the plane in time! Because I'm at home, not having my suitcase has not been a major problem but for tourists arriving in a foreign country without their luggage it is a much bigger problem. I'm surprised that my travel agent who booked the flight from Stockholm to Heathrow didn't realise that two hours to change terminals and connect with another flight is not enough time at Heathrow.

On Monday afternoon I visit the doctor who completed the medical declaration for my application for travel insurance to cover an existing condition. *They declined my application, I appealed but they still declined. But I didn't need any medical assistance while I was away* I tell him. "I'm not surprised, but you got away with it" he says. I still don't think it is fair. Why should people be denied insurance cover for an existing condition? Companies could charge an increased premium based on the risk. There must be plenty of people out there with, for example, heart disease, who would not have cover if they needed something like cardiac surgery or angioplasty while they are away. The majority of people would, like me, not need to make a claim while they are away, but the cover would be there for those who need it and are prepared to pay the premium.

14

Learning to be patient - September 2006

Over the last few months, in my capacity as Asia-Pacific study manager for a global stent registry, I have been reviewing site selection audit reports for hospitals in China and Taiwan. The audits have been conducted by Judy, a Taiwanese CRA working in our sister company in Japan. I reply to an email from Judy's manager:

> I'm finding it interesting and I'm only sorry that I can't do some of the audits myself!! – 2 reasons 1) can't speak Chinese 2) can't speak period!

> She replies:

> Aaah, Barb! How is your health these days? Your positive spirits are truly amazing!

And I elaborate:

> I'm OK – it's getting harder but I'm hanging in there!

I am hanging in there, but it is getting harder. I have never been a patient person. I've always been in a hurry to do things and now everything takes longer. I'm learning to be patient. Although it's frustrating, I'm fairly relaxed about things. I guess it's a case of having to be - I'd go mad otherwise.

Even the ordinary everyday things that we all take for granted are difficult. My fingers have lost their fine dexterity and I have trouble doing up buttons. Because my fingers won't grasp the tab on the zipper on my trousers I have tied little ribbon loops onto the tabs. I can just slip my finger into the loop and pull up the zip. I no longer wear earrings because I can't get the post through the hole in my earlobe. I've stopped wearing eye makeup because the mascara runs when I cry. Similarly lipstick doesn't last long because I'm continually biting my lips in a constant battle to control excess saliva.

Cutting my nails is hard because I can't hold the nail scissors in my left hand. Even holding scissors in my right hand I don't have the strength to cut through thick nails. Drying my back after a shower isn't easy either.

Because I don't have the full range of movement with my left hand when undressing I have trouble getting my left arm out of the sleeve of a cardigan or coat. I struggle to pull t-shirts over my head and it can take several attempts to finally get the t-shirt off.

In my tiny one-bedroom apartment I need to stop and rest halfway through vacuuming the floor. When I wash my sheets I have trouble putting the duvet back on my bed as it's too heavy for me to lift. When peeling potatoes I fumble with the peeler. I have difficulty getting hot and heavy cookware out of the oven. I need to bend down, grab the container with both hands and then somehow stand up without spilling or dropping anything.

I have to travel with all the 'gear' that I need. My checked-in suitcase and my carry-on bags are heavier now and yet I'm less able to manage them. I can no longer lift bags up to put them in the overhead locker in the plane. Recently after struggling to hoist my backpack up into the overhead locker I give up in frustration and throw the backpack down with some force on to the seat. A young lady behind me offers to put the bag up for me. I shake my head "I'm serious, I'll do it" she says so, feeling sheepish I pass the bag to her. Unable to say "thank you" I smile and give her the 'thumbs up'. Another time on an evening flight from Brisbane to Sydney a man seeing me struggle puts my backpack up for me. The man is sitting in the row in front of me and when we arrive in Sydney he gets my backpack down and carries it off the plane for me while I pull my computer bag along behind me.

Until recently I have been able to utter an understandable "thanks" but now I can't even do that. I feel awful. There are so many times in the course of a day that you want to say "thanks." In the supermarket or shop, to taxi drivers, when someone holds the door open etc. The other day as I am coming in the main entrance of the apartment building where I live, a young boy standing on the inside of the glass entry door opens it for me. With hands full of shopping and mail I can't give him the 'thumbs up' and I just keep on walking. The boy's dad who is in the process of unlocking his ground floor apartment door says "Thank you," and when I don't reply he says to his son "She should say thank you." In another situation I would have stopped, flashed my *I've lost my voice* card and indicated my gratitude, but I regularly hear this man shouting abusively at his son or the dog and I always try to avoid him when I can.

The PEG tube has made things easier. Taking medication is no longer something to be dreaded. I take most fluids via the tube because I can only swallow one or two very small sips of water. When I'm eating a meal I can still drink water or Coke. It seems that the action of chewing and swallowing food relaxes things making it easier to swallow fluids. I can't swallow other 'sodas' but Coke goes down easily; maybe it's the pH of Coke that makes it easier to drink. I can usually still eat breakfast of porridge, or bacon, hash browns and poached egg, or pancakes with lots of maple syrup. I try to have one can of Jevity via the tube at about 11am and another at 2pm or if I'm busy I'll have both cans at once at about mid day. I will usually eat something soft for dinner.

I'm getting used to taking medication or Jevity via the tube in all sorts of public places. At the airport, waiting for a flight in the Qantas Club often I find a fairly private spot in the business centre. On planes I just get on with it in my seat and try to ignore everyone around me. Sometimes I'm lucky to have an empty seat beside me, other times I have one or more people beside me. Some of my experiences have been mentioned earlier. During the cruise I just got on with it, having a can of Jevity or my medication via the tube while on the bus or at a streetside café. I need to be organised though. I carry my 50ml syringe, pill crusher, small plastic pots (for dissolving the medication) plastic fork (for stirring) and teaspoon (for levering up the pull tab on the can of Jevity). I keep all this in a small plastic container so all I need to do is pop the lid on and go. I also need to carry a bottle of water, one or two cans of Jevity and my medication. With all of this and a book and reading glasses my backpack is quite heavy.

For some months I have noticed that my left leg has a bluish tinge after I have been sitting for a while. I wonder if my leg is ischemic but I have no particular risk factors for arterial disease and I'm not a smoker. The pulses in my leg and foot are OK. I wonder if it is caused by some sort of arterial constriction when I'm sitting or maybe my blood gases are so bad that my skin looks cyanosed. I've been waiting to have my blood gases measured for a couple of months now but every time I visit the respiratory clinic they don't have the right blood tube for the test. For several months I've noticed grey spots on two toes and in the first week in July I noticed a blister on my left heel which has not healed and at times it is quite painful. However, I carry on with my busy schedule and I don't take much notice of it.

During the week before I leave for the Baltic cruise my left ankle is swollen by the end of the day but after a night in bed the swelling goes away. During the cruise I notice that my left foot is swollen and one day my left leg is swollen right up to the knee. My left foot and leg up to mid calf or knee is quite blue/purple after standing in the shower. It's really quite frightening. Luckily I have some elastic stockings with me, having planned to wear them in the plane, and I start wearing one on my left leg during the day and when possible I elevate my leg while I'm sitting.

Back home after the trip I start wondering what the matter is. Then it occurs to me that maybe because I've lost muscle in my left leg, it's venous pooling. I do a quick internet search and sure enough the answer is there.

Veins need the muscles in our feet and legs to help the blood return, against gravity, to the heart. Venous pooling can occur when there is no musculoskeletal pump in the legs. This causes swelling in the legs, changes in skin colour, enlargement of the veins close to the surface of the skin and skin ulcers, usually on or near the ankle. Treatment to reduce the pooling of blood and to help prevent ulcers includes elevation of the legs to allow pooled blood to drain and compression of veins close to the skin by wearing elastic stockings to prevent pooling.[1]

I'm wearing an elastic stocking on my left leg every day but it is very hard to pull on, especially now that my fingers are losing their strength. I have bought a plastic hosiery donning aid. The stocking is fed on to the plastic tube then the foot is put in the open end of the stocking, which is then pulled over the foot and up the leg using tapes on the side of the plastic tube. Simple in theory but the process takes me about five minutes each morning.

I eventually get to see the occupational therapist. She takes baseline measurements of the range of my hand/finger movements. Next she shows me how to do the finger, thumb and wrist exercises and she asks me to do them twice a day. She also gives me some Thera Putty, a sort of play dough for me to roll out in to a long thin strip with my weak left fingers. Home I go and set about doing the exercises. To do them properly takes me the best part of 30 minutes twice a day. Getting time to do the exercises when I'm away from home will be difficult, especially if I'm on a day trip to Melbourne or Brisbane. *I could roll out the Thera Putty on the tray table in the plane* I think. But I immediately realise that in this era of airline terrorism that wouldn't be such a good idea. *They will think I'm a terrorist rolling out plastic explosive! Maybe I can just do the other exercises. People will think I'm mad but they probably do anyway when I can't talk.*

A week later I go back to see the occupational therapist. She shows me other things to do that will increase the dexterity of my left thumb and index finger. My right hand is starting to show signs of muscle loss so I also need to do exercises with my right hand.

I wonder why it was that I needed to ask to be referred for hand therapy, just as I had to ask whether a night-time resting splint would be helpful. Surely a rehabilitation specialist should have examined all of the areas of potential difficulty such as hands, feet and legs, and pro-actively initiated therapy. For that matter, why wasn't this considered a year or so ago at the MND clinic?

I've only been back from Europe for just over one week when I get an email from Kevin telling me that Barbara's father Bob has died. Her mother, Betty, died earlier in the year. I make plans to travel to Christchurch for the funeral. Using my frequent flyer points I'm able to get a return ticket to Christchurch on the Qantas holiday airline Jet Star.

Thursday morning comes and I'm up early. I phone the taxi. The taxi phone's recorded message has changed now and the first question is "What is the name of the suburb that you are travelling to?" I say "airport" but the automatic machine does not understand me. After several attempts to say "airport" I'm transferred to an operator. The operator can't understand me either. After several attempts we settle on Enmore as the suburb that I'm going to and I go downstairs hoping that the taxi will arrive. The taxi arrives as I'm coming out the front door and I'm on my way.

Arriving at the airport I go to the Qantas Club check in counter only to be told that I need to check in at the Jet Star counter at the other end of the departures terminal. Fortunately there isn't a queue and I'm checked in fairly quickly. The Jet Star flight departs from gate 63 which is in the other section of the international terminal to where the Qantas Club lounge is located. I had been hoping to check my emails in the Qantas Club but I realise that I won't have enough time to do this and walk along to gate 63, so I just go straight to the gate and wait to board.

The plane is a fairly new Airbus with orange trim. Only about a quarter of the seats are occupied so it's a comfortable flight. The cabin crew are dressed as though they are working in a holiday camp and the passengers need to pay for all extras including food and drink. This suits me though as I have a can of Jevity, a bottle of water and I won't be eating. I also travel with my own earphones.

In Christchurch Barbara asks if I would like to be a pall bearer and my initial response is "no." However, we talk about it and I realise that I will be able to manage with my right hand if I'm in the middle and I agree to be a pall bearer. Bob had been in the Navy during the war, the Naval White Ensign is on the coffin, the hymn *Eternal Father* (for those in peril on the sea) is sung, a man from the RSA speaks and the Naval version of the "Last Post" is played. Bob had a wonderful sense of humour and a brilliant turn of phrase and in her eulogy Barbara recounts many wonderful memories. The funeral is a fitting tribute to Bob's life, and not really a sad occasion as Bob, having suffered from Alzheimer's disease for the last few years, is now at peace with his wife Betty. Yet I find it distressing, and have several tearful moments during the service. It's just too much of a reminder of what is going to happen to me.

I spend a quiet weekend in Christchurch with Barbara and her friend Robyn. The sunny spring weather, blossoms on the trees and daffodils in the park framed by the snow covered mountains in the distance is Christchurch at its best. Sunday afternoon I'm back on the holiday airline and on my way back to Sydney.

Shortly after arriving back from Christchurch I return to the respiratory clinic for a 'nap' mask fitting test. Following another uncomfortable sleep test and more lung function tests in June and July the doctor and I had both agreed that I wouldn't start using overnight BiPAP until I returned from the cruise in August.

The technician fits the mask, then she turns the BiPAP machine on and leaves the room shutting the door. She gives me no instructions and doesn't check that I am comfortable. The mask has two small soft bulbs (cushions) that sit at the entrance to the nostrils. In theory it should be good, delivering air directly into the nose but I don't find it that comfortable and air leaks out of my mouth.

After about half an hour the technician returns and takes the mask off and I wait for the doctor to come and see me. The doctor again discusses my need for overnight non-invasive ventilation and we agree that although my need is not urgent it is a good idea to give it a go. In his words "it's thought that ventilation gives your breathing muscles a rest overnight and they might not wear out so quickly." He gives me a prescription for the machine and tells me that I will need to pick it up from the supplier.

It takes about two weeks to get set up at home with the machine and mask. The machine is actually VPAP (variable positive airways pressure) not BiPAP, although I'm not sure what the difference is.

I start using the mask and machine. I can go to sleep easily but there is a fine art to getting the mask on properly so it doesn't leak. I alternate between two different masks. The mask that has the cushions that sit over the nostrils gets uncomfortable and I find that I can only tolerate it for a few hours then I need to swap to the mask that covers the whole nose. This mask is more comfortable but it leaks around my top lip. By 5am when I have my Riluzole I usually leave the mask off for the rest of the night.

Compliance is a big issue with home-based overnight non-invasive ventilation and from my own experience I have found this to be true. With the best will in the world, and being acutely aware from my reading of medical journals that starting non-invasive ventilation early is associated with better survival, I am finding it difficult to keep the mask on all night. Also there is no way that I will be able to travel regularly with the VPAP machine. It's just too heavy for me to manage along with my other carry on luggage.

I am having increasing difficulty calling taxis. Sometimes at hospitals the 'taxi' phone by the main entrance is automated so that you only have to respond to the prompts by pressing one number. For example the message goes something like "If you want a taxi for three or less people and are ready now press 1." Other times you have to say the name of the suburb that you are travelling to. One time at Fremantle Hospital I ask the lady at the reception desk if she will call a taxi for me. I overhear her saying "I have a lady here who is mute ...." I know that I can't speak but I don't like being referred to as 'mute.' The word mute conjures up images of disability. I would rather she had used the term "lost her voice."

At about this time my social worker sends me some information about the National Relay Service (NRS). This is a telephone service for people who can't hear or speak clearly. Using a special phone the call goes through a relay officer who 'relays' the voice or text to the other person and vice versa. So with help from my social worker and my speech therapist I submit an application to use this service. In due course my application is accepted and the teletypewriter phone arrives by registered post. It's a compact phone with a typewriter keyboard and a small display screen. It's easily installed and within days I'm using it to call taxis.

Quite some time ago someone mentioned this service to me but the information about it was vague and I never followed it up. However, the system is so easy to use that I wonder why I didn't follow it up earlier. The instruction booklet that comes with the phone has quite clear instructions for making and receiving calls with text, in other words for non-hearing people. However, the instructions for 'hearing carry over calls,' where I type my message and hear the other person speaking their response, are very vague. I find that it's easier and quicker to pretend I'm deaf and send and receive messages in text. This works fine for calling taxis.

I'm on my way to Auckland on a LAN Chile flight. Lunch is a toasted chicken and cheese sandwich. I ask for a glass of coke. Usually on Qantas flights I have no problems drinking a glass of coke. However, on this plane the glass is much wider than those on the Qantas planes. I pick up the glass in my (good) right hand. The glass promptly slips out of my hand and my attempts to rescue the glass only serve to send the glass and contents into my lap!! *Oh no!* I think. Fortunately the man sitting beside me calls out to the cabin attendant "Can we have some serviettes please?" I clean myself up and then write a note to the man. Thanks, I've lost my voice. For the rest of the flight I sit there with wet pants. A little later I get up and walk to the toilet - the wet patch looks like I have wet my pants. Luckily it's dry by the time we get to Auckland and I have another pair of trousers to wear for my monitoring visits.

On Wednesday the following week I'm on my way to Christchurch. I realise that I won't be able to eat either the pasta or the curried lamb for lunch so I ask the flight attendant to get my backpack down and while everyone else is eating their lunch I have two tins of Jevity followed by my lunchtime tablet. The plane is full, I am sitting in my forward aisle seat near the galley, and the surrounding passengers and the cabin crew all have a good view of proceedings. As we are descending into Christchurch I ask the same flight attendant to put my backpack back up in the overhead locker. "Do you need help to get through customs?" she asks. I shake my head indicating no.

Maybe I should have accepted the assistance offered. With walking stick in hand I hobble along the 'families with children/disabled' lane hoping it will be quicker. But it isn't! The passport lady looks at every page in my passport. They don't usually do this. *What's the matter?* I wonder. I collect my suitcase from the baggage carousel and head towards the agricultural x-ray. The screening officer looks at my arrivals card and directs me to a customs officer, not, as usually happens, to the x-ray machine. *What is going on?* I wonder. The customs lady asks me to follow her. She asks me to sit in an alcove and she takes my passport away. When she comes back she says she wants to search my bags. I write WHY? "You fit a profile" she says. *Sure I fit a profile* I think *I'm a middle aged woman who can't speak and can hardly walk!*

"Why do you travel so much?' She asks. I show her my business card and write travel to hospitals in AU & NZ. "I'll go and speak to my supervisor" she says. When she comes back she says "I'll need to look in one of your bags" and she dons a pair of rubber gloves and starts to search my suitcase. She picks up the plastic container of Thera Putty, takes a look at the label and puts it on the pile with the rest of my things. I've already mentioned the contents of my tins of Jevity to her and when she comes to the eight tins in the bottom of my case I show her my letter from the dietician at St George Hospital verifying my need for Jevity.

Finding nothing suspicious she re-packs my bag commenting on how neatly everything is packed. Then she leads me to the head of the x-ray queue and loads my bags onto the conveyer. "Thank you for co-operating" she says. In all the time I've been travelling I've never been questioned or searched like this before. I'm hardly a prime suspect for a drug runner!

I have two uneventful days monitoring at Christchurch hospital and on Friday afternoon I take a taxi to Barbara's place where I'm staying for the weekend. Later in the afternoon I realise that the taxi driver didn't enter the price on the American Express payment slip that I signed. Barbara phones the taxi company and explains the situation. The taxi lady is able to tell Barbara the number of the taxi and says that she will ring back with the price. I know roughly how much the trip cost so we will be able to challenge any inflated price. Despite ringing back several times during the weekend they still can't tell Barbara the cost of the taxi fare. It seems that they are stalling. I return to Sydney and Barbara says that she will keep on calling the taxi company.

On Saturday morning we drive to Lyttelton and get the ferry over to Diamond Harbour. It's a sunny day but there is a strong north westerly wind. Getting off the ferry we see a sign saying 'café' and pointing to a track up the hill. So off we go up the cliff via concrete steps, a stony path and more steps all heading up hill. I need to stop and rest a couple of times while Barbara goes on ahead to see if we are nearly there. By the time we realise that we have been climbing for a while and Barbara still can't see the café, we decide that it's easier to keep going than to go back down and walk up the road. Luckily I have my walking stick. I would not have managed without it. Eventually we get to the cafe and sit down at an outside table. I'm exhausted. I feel like a frail old lady. We look at the menu but it's pretty uninspiring and we decide to get the ferry back to Lyttelton and have lunch there. So we go back down hill via the road. This is much easier than the up hill climb.

Back in Lyttelton Barbara hurries on ahead to get her car and bring it closer so that I don't have so far to walk and I struggle to climb the steps over the railway line. The wind is so strong that I have to hold on tight to the railing so I don't get blown over.

The rest of the weekend passes quietly. We watch two movies on DVD, *Mississippi Burning* and *A Beautiful Mind*. They are both movies that the kids have to write essays on in exams and Barbara is just about to start marking exam papers. Barbara says the kids have to write about production and lighting etc in the movies. I'd write about the ethical issues, I tell her.

On Saturday night Barbara watches the Kiwi/Lions rugby league game and then on Sunday morning she watches the All Blacks/ France rugby game. I read my book glancing up to see the exciting bits. Sunday afternoon I'm on my way back home to Sydney. I have no problems with customs in Sydney, I pass straight through the screening to the exit, no agricultural x-ray, there is no queue for the taxi and I arrive home 30 minutes after landing.

On Wednesday the following week I travel to Perth. My usual hotels are fully booked so I've taken pot luck choosing a hotel based on price, a restaurant and room service. On arrival at the hotel I am faced with a flight of steps up to the front door! While I'm wondering *Why do hotels have steps leading up to the front door?* I try unsuccessfully to attract the attention of the receptionist. Then I attempt to carry my bags up one at a time but I can't even make it up the first step with the first bag. My arms and legs are too weak to support the weight of the bag and climb the stairs at the same time. By now the receptionist has looked up, and seeing my plight she comes to the rescue.

Once checked in I take the elevator to the seventh floor. I try the key in the door to my room. I can't get the key to turn and open the door. I try again and again and again. Then, giving up, I write a note and leaving my bags by the door I go down to the receptionist. I can't get the key to open the door. "I'll come up and open it," she says, probably thinking that I'm hopeless. However, she struggles to get the door open too so I don't feel so bad.

Before she leaves I ask her about the hotel's restaurant as I noticed that the restaurant has a 'closed for renovations' sign on the door. When I booked on the internet I was careful to choose a hotel with a restaurant I tell her. What can I do for meals? I ask. "Our other hotel has a restaurant" she says. "It's a five minute walk." I can't walk that far. I tell her and pull up my trouser leg to show her my AFO. I'm here for 3 days - this is hopeless. I say and start to sob out of absolute frustration. I just can't believe this is happening.

I continue writing I travel every week for work – always book with a restaurant and room service. What can I do? I can't eat much. I pull up my shirt and show her my PEG tube. I manage very well in hotels with room service. This is HOPELESS. Where I usually stay is fully booked. I keep up the written tirade. "Would you like me to see if there is a room in our other hotel? She asks. I nod yes. "I'll go down and phone and come back and let you know" she says.

She returns. "There is a room. The taxi will take you there and the reception at the other hotel will pay for the taxi." Thanks! I write. She carries my bags down to the taxi. I'm sure she is breathing a sigh of relief to be rid of me!

At the next hotel they are expecting me and I'm quickly checked in. Key in hand I go up in the elevator to the second floor. Again I have trouble turning the key in the lock. I have a square of rubberised mesh in my bag that gives me a better grip on slippery surfaces. So after several attempts I get my 'grip' out of my bag and this does the trick, the door opens.

The hotel room is an older style fairly basic room. There is no remote for the TV, no drinking glass, no shower cap, no broadband connection, but at least there is a restaurant and room service.

The next morning the hotel receptionist calls a taxi for me and I'm outside waiting on the kerb for the cab. After a few minutes a taxi pulls up and I show the driver my note: Taxi to Fremantle Hospital main entrance Alma St. (name) Williams.

The driver shakes his head and drives away. And I wait. There are several other people waiting too. After about 20 minutes I'm still waiting. I go back inside and ask the receptionist to call the taxi again. While I'm doing this a taxi pulls up and one of the ladies who is waiting jumps in the cab. I rush down the steps and wave my note at the driver who only shakes his head and drives off with the lady in his cab. "She took your taxi" the other lady tells me. By now I have been waiting half an hour and I'm getting very frustrated. I start to cry from the utter hopelessness of the situation. Another taxi pulls up and waving my note at the driver I hop in before anyone else beats me to it. I'm still crying. The driver probably thinks I'm mad, but never mind. I eventually arrive at the hospital and get on with my work.

At the end of the day I go to the hospital's inquiries desk with my note *I've lost my voice. Please phone me a taxi*.........I wait out on the street for about 15 minutes before the taxi arrives. Once in the cab the driver asks me how I am going to pay. He thinks that I'm a patient with a taxi voucher. Once I show him my credit card he is happy and off we go. On Friday I have a bit more luck with taxis to and from the hospital arriving fairly promptly. I finish my work in good time and I spend the evening quietly in my hotel room writing my reports.

On Saturday morning I check out of the hotel. *Can you please call me a taxi to the airport and help me down the steps with my bags?* I ask. "I'll take your bags down in a minute" the receptionist says. As I move over to the door I can see that she is busy attending to other people. I carry my lightest bag down the steps without much trouble. Next I carry my heavy computer bag laboriously down one step at a time. With both bags safely on the footpath I bend over one to put something in the outside pocket of the other. Somehow I catch my foot on one of the bags and over I go. I feel like I'm falling in slow motion but there is nothing that I can do to stop the fall. I land sort of sideways on my bottom and I'm cast. I can't get up. Two people offer me a hand each and pull me back up on to my feet. Feeling silly I give them the thumbs up by way of thanks. Nothing seems to be broken or damaged. Just then the taxi arrives and I'm on my way to the airport for my trip back to Sydney.

The week before I had a similar fall while monitoring at a Brisbane Hospital. When I stood up and turned to get something out of my bag I caught my foot on the corner of my bag, lost my balance and slowly slipped to the floor. I'm beginning to feel quite unstable on my feet. All my life I have wandered around at home barefooted in summer and in slippers in winter. Now, I need to wear shoes and my AFO all the time to stop me falling. Without the AFO the toes on my left foot catch on the carpet and over I go.

At about this time I am saddened to read in the *New Zealand Herald* (on line) that Willie Terpstra, the lady who went to China for stem cell treatment, has died, roughly three years after being diagnosed with MND. I mention this in an email to a medical colleague who replies:

> The Terpstra news is sad indeed and not easy for you – but everyone including you is unique and time courses vary.

I do know that time courses for MND vary. I've been so good for so long, and I'm grateful for the time that I have had but now things are getting harder and I wonder how much time I have left. There are still lots of things that I want to achieve.

Two days later I'm on my way to Auckland. As I'm going to be away from home for ten days I've packed 20 tins of Jevity in a small backpack. I've also packed a copy of my Jevity letter from the dietician explaining my need to carry Jevity and certifying its agricultural safety. The bag of Jevity travels as checked in luggage because it's too heavy for me to carry as cabin baggage. On arrival in Auckland my suitcase and the bag of Jevity arrive side by side on the baggage carousel. I load them on my trolley and proceed past the customs man to the agricultural x-ray. Approaching the x-ray machine I indicate to the man that I would like some help with my bags. He places my suitcase on the belt and says "You can do it, they aren't heavy." My suitcase is much lighter than my computer bag or my bag of Jevity so I just look dumbly at him until he has loaded the bags. The bags pass through the x-ray machine and sure enough they stop my bag of Jevity. "What are all the tins?" the man asks starting to open the bag. I show him my *I've lost my voice* notice and putting my hand in the bag I pull out my Jevity letter. He reads the letter and says "That's OK" and I'm free to go.

For the next nine days I have a hectic schedule. I'm at the new Auckland City Hospital on Wednesday. Thursday morning I'm up at 5am and off to Wellington on an early flight and back to Auckland in the afternoon. On Friday I collect a rental car and drive to Waikato hospital in Hamilton.

On the way back from Hamilton to Auckland I stop at Ngaruawahia. There is a strip of grass between the main highway and the railway line. People in trucks and buses and cars stop here to eat lunch and use the toilets. I unload my backpack from the car and step backwards on to the grass verge. My heel catches the concrete kerb and I fall down flat on my bottom. I'm not hurt and I pull myself up, make my way to one of the picnic tables and have two cans of Jevity for lunch. Shortly a tour bus stops across the road and the Japanese tourists cross the road and walk past me to the toilet block. I feel several of them staring at me as they pass but I continue to gaze off into the distance holding my syringe of Jevity high in the air.

Arriving back in Auckland I pop in to visit my former colleagues at the old Green Lane Hospital, now called the Greenlane Clinical Centre, before returning the rental car and getting a taxi home to Birkenhead.

I have a quiet Saturday catching up on sleep and work. On Sunday we have a BBQ lunch for Dylan and my birthdays. Most of the extended family are there and it's a lovely sunny day. We spend a leisurely and very enjoyable afternoon on the deck in the sun. I manage to eat one sausage and I enjoy it so much that I ask Kevin to cook me another on the BBQ for dinner.

Monday morning I'm up at 5am again to get the early flight to Dunedin. Although the plane is a Boeing 737 there are steps up to the plane, not an air bridge. As I'm boarding the plane I show the cabin attendant my note *I've lost my voice. I need help to get my bag up the steps.* "Leave it here and I'll bring it" she says. She keeps my note and writes my seat number on it.

I start to climb the steps up to the plane. The first step is quite high off the ground and placing my left foot on the step, holding the hand rail I pull myself up. My left leg collapses under me and it is all I can do to stop falling. Somehow I recover my balance and slowly pull myself up the steps.

Once in the air I have breakfast. At home I emptied two boxes of Sanitarium *Up & Go* liquid Weetbix into a bottle and sitting in my window seat with two people sitting beside me, I pull out my syringe and get on with it.

As we are descending in to Dunedin the cabin attendant asks if I will need help with my bag. I write *If air bridge Ok - if steps will need help.* Even though there is an air bridge at the new Dunedin terminal the plane stops on the tarmac and steps are pulled up to the door. Next I'm faced with a staircase up to the arrivals floor in the terminal. Fortunately one of the Air New Zealand ground staff carries my computer bag up the stairs for me while, holding the hand rail, I slowly pull myself up the stairs. Once on the top level of the terminal I'm faced with a choice of the escalator or the elevator to get down to the ground floor baggage claim area. I choose the elevator. It's crazy. Why can't passengers arriving on the tarmac walk straight though to the baggage claim without having to needlessly go up and down?

After a day at Dunedin Hospital I get a taxi out to Sawyers Bay where I'm spending the night with Barbara and her friend Robyn. Robyn lives in a lovely sunny house at Sawyers Bay and Barbara has been staying with her. It's December 4th, my 55th birthday, and after dinner Robyn brings out a cake with two groups of five candles. Barbara and Robyn sing 'Happy Birthday' but I'm not able to blow out the candles so they do it for me.

Next morning Barbara and I travel back to Christchurch together on the same plane. Having Barbara with me is great. She carries my heavy computer bag up the steps to the plane. It's a small ART72 propeller plane so the steps are more manageable for me but I still struggle. "Well done!" the male cabin attendant says as I reach the top.

I have an uneventful day at Christchurch Hospital. In the late afternoon I travel by taxi to the hotel. My usual hotel was fully booked so I've chosen a different one based on my usual criteria of price, restaurant, room service and internet access. Seeing me struggle with my luggage trying to get through the revolving door, the porter comes and helps me. Once I've checked in, the porter accompanies me to my room bringing my luggage.

I've been upgraded to a two bedroom apartment on the 26th floor. There is a spectacular view, towards the east, of the Port Hills and suburban Christchurch. The striking thing is the sea of green trees stretching all the way to the Pacific Ocean. Exploring the apartment I carefully pull myself up the stairs to have a look at the loft bedroom. The wooden stairs are steep and I'm very conscious of the consequences of a fall down these stairs. Needless to say I choose to sleep in the downstairs bedroom.

At 6pm with note in hand I go down to the restaurant to order a room service dinner. As usual my note starts off :

I've lost my voice. I would like room service. Followed by my choice of meal and signed off with my name and room number.

Handing my note to the waitress she remarks "What a good way to do it. No problems. It will be about 30 minutes."

Returning to my room I put the key in the door. I can't get the key to turn. After several unsuccessful attempts I give up and go back down to the ground floor to get some help. I see the porter who helped me with my luggage and indicate that I want to write something. I can't open my door. I show him my left hand which with stiffened fingers is becoming claw-like. "No problem" he says as we walk to the elevator. Soon I'm back in my room and before long I'm enjoying tender stuffed chicken breast, cheesy baked potatoes and a glass of coke.

On Wednesday morning I spend a couple of hours at Christchurch Hospital before heading to the airport for my flight back to Sydney. As I pass through the customs check point the lady flicks through the pages of my passport. "You have a lot of travel in here" she says but fortunately she doesn't pull me out for closer questioning.

Once in the Qantas Club I head to the business centre to check my emails. All the computers are in use so I sit down in the main lounge area and have two cans of Jevity for lunch. In full view of everyone in the lounge I'm holding the syringe high in the air and staring into the distance. I try to ignore the glances of the other passengers. When it is time to board the plane I re-pack my book and glasses in my computer bag. As I'm bending over the bag I hear someone saying "Hello, hello." Not realising that the man is talking to me I continue packing my bag. Then looking up I see that the man is talking to me. "Would you like me to carry your bag for you?' he asks. I shake my head. "Are you sure?" he asks and I shake my head again. I can very easily manage to wheel my computer bag on to the plane if there is an air bridge. I would have liked to thank the man for his kindness but with my paper packed away the opportunity passes.

Later in the plane after eating my lunch (I'm only able to manage the pieces of braised pork, I can't manage the rice or peas) I struggle to hold my tray up, close my tray table and get up from my seat to go to the toilet. In the past I've done this effortlessly many times. But this time I'm struggling. The lady in the seat across the aisle holds out her hand to take my tray. She places it on her tray table while I get up from my seat. I smile and give her the thumbs up. Again I am touched by the kindness shown to me by a total stranger.

Arriving back in Sydney the airport is quiet, I clear immigration and customs quickly and before long I'm home. I'm absolutely exhausted and a bit disorientated. I usually come back to Sydney from New Zealand on a Sunday night and it's only Wednesday. Later I email Robyn to thank her for having me to stay. She replies:

> I'm not surprised you're tired. I would find even coping with the weather and temperature variations in all the different centres tiring, let alone the work itself. Personally, I reckon you're pretty amazing....

Amazing or selfish? I wonder. I have been stubbornly determined to carry on for as long as I can but it is getting harder.

1 *Chronic Venous Insufficiency. Information for you and your health care team.* SUNY Upstate Medical University. http://www.upstate.edu/uhpated/pdf/chronic_venous_insuff.pdf

15

Sadly the time has come - December 2006

I have been stubbornly determined to carry on for as long as I can. Sadly, though, the time has come that I have to stop doing site visits as a CRA. Over the last few months travelling and everything else has been getting much more difficult.

It's the week before Christmas and I'm in Melbourne for four days finishing off a marathon round of monitoring visits that in the last couple of months have taken me to all of my sites in both Australia and New Zealand.

I spend uneventful days at The Alfred Hospital on Monday and at Monash Medical Centre on Tuesday. On Monday night I choose 'grilled snapper with hand cut chips' for my room service dinner. When my meal arrives the snapper is accompanied by rocket salad, which I can't eat, but no chips. However, the snapper is so delicious that on Tuesday evening I order the same. This time I specifically ask for hand cut chips and state on my note no salad. My meal duly arrives. On the tray is a plate with snapper and a handful of chips and on the side a tinfoil covered bowl of chips. I shake my head in disbelief and start eating. The fish isn't as nice as yesterday's fish - it's probably a day older! I can't finish the chips on my plate let alone eat any of the extra chips in the bowl. When I'm finished I write a note to the kitchen staff and leave it on my tray outside my room:

> I've lost my voice.
>
> I have motor neurone disease and I can't eat many foods.

> On the room service menu is: Grilled snapper, hand cut chips $26.00.
>
> Last night, 18 Dec, the grilled snapper arrived with salad, NO chips.
>
> So tonight I asked for grilled snapper AND hand cut chips.
>
> What was delivered to my room was grilled snapper, chips on the plate AND a bowl of chips and coke total cost $40.00.
>
> Where am I/you going wrong?
>
> B Williams Room 2102.

Next morning I'm off to Box Hill Hospital for the day. With my back pack slung over my right shoulder and pulling my computer bag along I'm holding my left hand up to hail a taxi parked in the 'only in Melbourne' middle of the road taxi stand. At the same time I step down the two steps from the hotel to the footpath. Next thing I'm sitting on my bottom on the pavement. As I stepped off the step, weighed down by my bags, my legs collapsed under me and I guess I was concentrating on hailing the taxi rather than on walking down the steps. A man standing on the foot path turns to look at me and I hold out my hand to him. He pulls me up to my feet and by now the taxi has pulled up at the kerb. I'm on my way out to Box Hill, not hurt but feeling a little silly.

In the evening, back at the hotel, I go down to the restaurant to order my room service meal. I'm not going to risk having snapper again so I order chicken breast. Tonight a different waitress takes my order but my note must have had an impact. "Did someone phone you about last night's meal?" she asks. I shake my head. "They made a mistake and they have given you a credit on your account." I murmur my thanks and start to walk out of the restaurant. Another lady calls out "Mrs. Williams" I turn towards her. "Hello, I'm the food and beverages manager. The kitchen made a mistake with your meal last night. Please accept our apologies." Thanks Rydges Hotel!

Seemingly endless bush fires have been raging in the state of Victoria during December and on Wednesday the City of Melbourne is shrouded in a smoky haze. It's a bit like LA smog but grey/white, while I seem to remember that LA smog is a yellow/brown colour. I think it's a bit more low lying than LA smog and it's really eerie.

On Thursday morning I get up and walk to the window to check the weather. There is still smoke haze but it doesn't seem quite as bad as yesterday. Stepping back from the window I bang into the foot stool and over I go backwards, clonking my head on the floor. Fortunately the carpet cushions my fall and I'm not hurt.

I check out of the hotel and spend a couple of hours at St.Vincent's Hospital before heading to the airport and back to Sydney. I have 36 hours at home in Sydney to finish off my work and pack to be ready to go to Auckland for Christmas.

On Friday morning I email all of the people that I have been working with at the hospitals and sponsoring companies in the USA:

> Sadly, the time has come that I have to stop doing site visits as a CRA. I wish to thank all of you for your patience, support and friendship over these past couple of years.
>
> In January I will be handing over..................
>
> I will still retain an active interest in ....in the New Year in my new capacity as Research Manager.

These are a couple of the many lovely emails I receive throughout the day from colleagues:

> Thank you for conducting our site visit recently. I am saddened, as I'm sure the rest of the crew will be to hear we will no longer see you in person, but we do understand the enormous effort it must have taken you to move yourself from place to place with your increasing number/weight of bags!! It was a pleasure to know you, Barbara and I wish you all the very best in your new position. Hope you get some sunshine in Auckland over the Christmas break!

> This is so unfortunate, and I wish things were different! ....
> for me you serve as a symbol of how professionalism, excellence, dedication and courage can win everything against all odds! I admire you for not giving up and wishing you only the best!
> Thanks for the update and I love and admire your passion for work and life.

I am fortunate that I still have a job and that I can contribute to the company in a new role. I look forward to the challenge.

On Saturday morning I'm up at 4am. After a quick shower, I take my morning Riluzole tablet a little early and pack the last few things in my case. As I'm going to be in Auckland for about three weeks I've packed 36 cans of Jevity in a photocopy paper box and I have labelled it in the same way that I did when I went to London. I've also packed eight cans of Jevity in my suitcase. As well, I have my computer bag and my backpack, all of which are heavy. There is no way that I can take everything down to the taxi in one trip. I put the box of Jevity on my trolley and wheel it out to the elevator and down to the front door. It's 4:45 am and there is no one around, but just to be sure, I leave the box in full view of the security camera at the entrance to the building. Next I repeat the process with my suitcase. Then I phone for the taxi using the TTY phone – *this is so easy, why didn't I get it much sooner?* I wonder.

By the time I arrive at the front door the taxi is waiting. I show the driver my note Can you help with my bags please? And I point to the suitcase and box by the front door. Once we are in the taxi I show the driver my I've lost my voice card. "That is my church" he says pointing to the Greek church and we are on our way to the International Terminal.

Arriving at the terminal I pay the driver and hop out of the cab and walk over to the luggage trolleys. To release a trolley I need to put $4 into the machine. I have a $2 coin and two $1 coins in my hand. My hands won't grip the coins properly and I drop 2 of the coins as I'm feeding them into the machine. The dropped coins have vanished but luckily I have more coins in my purse and eventually I've fed enough coins into the machine and a trolley is released. Inside the terminal I go to the Qantas Business Class check in counter but there is no one there because I'm too early. I walk over to the next line of check in counters and join the long economy class queue. Just then I see a lady opening up the First Class check in counter so I leave the economy queue and walk over to the First Class counter. "I'm not open yet" the lady says and asks me if I'm travelling First Class. I show her my Business Class e-ticket and she says "OK just wait a few minutes, I open at 5:30."

Once I'm checked in I wait in the coffee shop for the international departure area to open at 6am. My plane is boarding at 7:05. I know that I am early but I'd rather be early than leave home later and have something go wrong and then have to rush. When I've cleared passport control and security I buy several last minute Christmas presents in the duty free shops and then it's time to board the plane to Auckland.

I got my plane ticket using my frequent flyer points and the only seat available before Christmas was in Business Class on this early flight. My preference would have been to travel later in the day or even on Sunday but it wasn't possible.

On the plane the breakfast service starts on the other aisle of the Business Class cabin and knowing how slowly the cabin crew serve the meals in Business Class I decide to have a can of Jevity while I'm waiting. I pour the Jevity into the syringe and hold it high. As the last of the Jevity is dripping through the flow stops. I can see that there are some globs of Jevity blocking the syringe. This has never happened before. *Did I forget to shake the can?* I wonder. I try to use the plunger to push it through but the black plastic bung on the end of the plunger has expanded and it won't fit in the end of the syringe. I want to tip the remaining Jevity out of the syringe. I really need a glass to tip it into but the cabin crew are still in the other aisle and I can't attract their attention so I tip it into the Jevity can. Big globby plugs of Jevity come out but the funnel end of the syringe is still blocked. I disconnect the syringe, poke the funnel end into the Jevity can and pour some water into the syringe. This does the trick but the PEG tubing is still blocked.

I place the end of the tubing over the Jevity can and lower it down hoping that gravity will allow some stomach contents to flow back up the tube and unblock it. This works. I still have time to crush my tablet and take it via the tube before my breakfast comes. I'm only able to eat the bacon and the yoke of the poached eggs so I'm glad that I had a can of Jevity.

Before long we land in Auckland. I pass through immigration, collect my suitcase and box of Jevity and proceed to the customs/agricultural screening point. "Do you have any food?" the man asks. I flash my *I've lost my voice* card and with a green felt marker he writes *Food? Fruit?* on a sheet of paper. He thinks I'm deaf, but I don't enlighten him, I just shake my head and he directs me to the agricultural x-ray. My bags and box of Jevity pass through the x-ray without further questioning. Kevin is waiting for me, we walk to the car and we are on our way home.

Kevin cooks roast pork for dinner, it's delicious and I'm able to eat the roast potatoes, pumpkin and kumera as well as the pork. I chomp away on the pork crackling too. Recently I've been losing weight steadily so I'm not concerned about eating 'naughty' foods such as pork crackling. So long as I can place food between the molars on my right side I can chew food well enough to be able to swallow it. This is easier than trying to swallow mushy food which seeps out through my lips.

On Sunday I do some last minute Christmas shopping and, apart from not having sent anyone Christmas cards, I'm ready for Christmas.

We have a quiet Christmas Day, despite there being 17 people, at my sister Jenni's house. I manage a slice of ham, some turkey and a small piece of pumpkin. Then I reach into my backpack and pull out the two cans of Jevity. I can't find my box of tricks (syringe etc). I've left them at home! I've been so busy collecting up all the presents etc. that I must have just missed packing the box. So on a day of traditional overeating I don't get enough to eat. It's at times like this that I really miss not being able to eat like everyone else.

I am staying in Auckland for three weeks but, having used up my annual leave days in August on the Baltic cruise, I spend most of the time at my computer working. Most of my work is conducted via email. Luckily my laptop computer can pick up a broadband connection via Kevin's network. The only problem I have is pulling myself up the steep stairs to the work area several times a day. The wooden handrail is flat rather than round and it's too wide for me to grip it properly. Because I'm scared of falling I take extra care and I'm painfully slow climbing the stairs one at a time. By the end of each day I'm exhausted.

On Saturday Kevin and I travel to Tauranga. We stay Saturday night with Kevin's brother Albert, his wife Dorothea and their daughter Tanya. On Sunday morning two of Kevin's cousins, Marie and Nita, come and visit and it's lovely to catch up with everyone.

We spend New Year's eve with Kevin's brother Brian and his wife Cecily at their house in Papamoa. I soak my feet in Cecily's foot spa and then Cecily gives me a foot massage which is really nice. Cecily who is a nurse in a retirement village notices my swollen left foot. *This leg has poor venous return coz no muscles* I tell her. Despite wearing a pressure stocking day and night, my left foot and ankle remain swollen.

Brian and Cecily spent three months in Europe this year. They went on a Baltic cruise that was similar to the one that Mum and I went on and I enjoy seeing the photos of their trip which brings back many happy memories of our cruise. We are all tired and we are in bed asleep before midnight. I have to work on January 2nd as it isn't a holiday in Australia so we head back to Auckland on New Year's day.

One evening, soon after we are back in Auckland, we go to Mum's new place for dinner. Her place in Takapuna was too cold in the winter so she has moved to a new apartment in a retirement village in Orakei. She has a wonderful view of Rangitoto and the gulf down towards Brown's Island with the Coromandel Peninsula in the distance. As the light fades the last rays of sun highlight Rangitoto. It looks so lovely.

The days pass in a flash and before long it's my last week in New Zealand. On Monday afternoon I travel to Christchurch. It's a lunch time flight and as the other passengers are eating their ham and cheese sandwich I have two cans of Jevity.

I get a taxi to Barbara's where I'm staying the night. In the evening we go to see the new James Bond film, *Casino Royale*, at the movies. As a teenager I read all of the James Bond books and saw many of the James Bond movies and this movie brings back memories. It's a good bit of escapism.

I'm up early on Tuesday morning and waiting at the end of the drive for Trish who is flying into Christchurch from Auckland. The taxi arrives and it's the same taxi driver who picked me up at the airport yesterday. I'm handing my studies over to Trish and we spend the day at Christchurch Hospital doing training and co-monitoring.

The study case report binders are heavy and I struggle to lift them, when six months ago I could handle them easily. I also struggle to turn the pages because my hands don't work properly. When I sign the site visit log there is a clear difference in my signature from earlier ones. Now my signature is shaky and spidery.

In the evening I return to Auckland. Low lying mist shrouds the airport and the plane is almost on the ground before we see the runway. I collect my luggage from the luggage carousel and head out to the taxi rank. There are four taxis waiting and the Indian taxi drivers are standing in a group talking. I show my driver my hand written address. He promptly has a discussion with the other drivers.The only word that I pick up is 'Onewa' so I guess he is asking how to get to Birkenhead.

We are on our way. Driving out of the airport the driver is hunched forward over the steering wheel gripping it tightly. It's a hot muggy night and before long the front window steams up. I'm sitting in the front passenger seat and I'm really tempted to reach over and turn the de-mister on. Before long it starts to rain. The driver turns the wipers on in the intermittent mode. As the rain gets harder the intermittent mode does not clear the windscreen quickly enough, but the driver doesn't turn the wipers to the continuous mode.

I open my window a little to let some cool air into the car. I am still tempted to reach over and turn the de-mister on and now I also want to turn the wipers to continuous. I don't do it, but I'm getting very frustrated. The driver is still hunched over the steering wheel and driving quite slowly. Eventually we get to my house and I pay the driver. He gets my bags out of the boot and starts to walk towards the front door with them. *Good* I think. But as he reaches the letter box he says "I'm keeping here." He drops the bags and heads back to his car. I start to pull my bags behind me and head down the short but fairly steep drive. I struggle and I nearly fall over. So one by one, I take the bags to the front door.

It's 9pm and Kevin is in bed asleep. I eat some ham for dinner and change into my nightie in the bathroom so I don't wake Kevin. Leaving my suitcase in the hallway I go to bed. I wake at 5am to take my Riluzole. It's still dark. Walking along the hallway to the bathroom I trip over my suitcase! Silly me, I knew it was there. I'm cast, spread-eagled across my suitcase. I slowly pull myself off the suitcase and pull myself over to a cupboard door. I grab the door handle and pull myself up. Not hurt, I go back to bed and sleep.

On Friday I get a taxi to Auckland City hospital where I meet Trish and we spend the day doing more training and co-monitoring. I've known Trish for many years and it doesn't matter that I can't speak. I communicate with her by writing notes. I use an old exercise book and by the end of our two days together I've filled up many pages. Once we are finished I say goodbye to Trish and head off to the Cardiology Department to say hello to several former colleagues. There is a new secretary. She doesn't know me and she asks me if I am a patient. I let her know that I'm a former staff member and before long I'm chatting to my old friends.

Afterwards while I'm making my way back along the corridor towards the elevator my right foot catches on the polished floor and I fall over. I'm not hurt but I can't get up by myself. A patient and a staff member come over to me and help me to my feet. I pick up my bag and start walking. Someone says "Come and sit down" but I keep going. I'm OK, this has happened before.

On Saturday Kevin goes off early to play bowls and I sleep in. Our friend Linda visits and we chat away with me writing down what I want to say. Linda has lunch and I have two cans of Jevity and then Linda drives me to the airport for my flight back to Sydney. In the Qantas 767 I have seats 24A and 24B to myself. Once the seat belt sign is off I get up to retrieve my backpack from the overhead locker. When I open the locker the Qantas bag of headphones falls out. I'm able to divert the fall with my arm and the bag lands harmlessly on the floor beside a lady sitting in 23A. The lady and the man sitting next to her look at me. I reach for my note pad and show them my *I've lost my voice* message written on the back of the pad and hope that they understand why I haven't said sorry.

I choose the chicken for lunch and I move over to sit in 24A so people can't see me using my fingers to manoeuvre the chicken around in my mouth. Then I have my two cans of Jevity. When I've finished lunch I move my tray to the empty seat and walk to the toilet. I'm sitting on the toilet when there is a frantic knocking on the toilet door. The person keeps knocking and knocking. I can't call out to ask what they want. I get up, do up my trousers and start washing my hands. The knocking continues and then the door starts to open. I push the door shut again and re-lock it. By the time I leave the toilet there is nobody there. I look around, everyone is sitting in their seats and there are no cabin attendants in sight. Shaking my head I walk back to my seat with no idea what the knocking was about.

It seems as though the three weeks in Auckland have passed in a flash and I'm back in Sydney for eight weeks before I move back to Auckland to live. It's getting harder to manage things on my own and once I'm no longer travelling for work I don't need to live in my 'close to the airport apartment.' My lease expires on March 6 and I want to be back in Auckland for Mum's 80th birthday on March 13.

Dylan is coming to Sydney for a week to help me move and we will both return to Auckland on Saturday March 10.

In the course of my work I email a colleague in California I haven't seen or heard from for a couple of years. In her response she mentions that her husband has a new job and isn't travelling any more. She says that:

> He doesn't really like having his wings clipped.

I respond:

> It's great to hear from you. The last 2 ½ years have been frantic and I have enjoyed every minute of it! My wings are clipped now too and I don't like it. But there isn't anything I can do about it – it's this bloody disease! I've got lots of interesting things to do though and I'm lucky to still be able to work. I'm moving back to Auckland on March 10 and I will continue working from there.

A few days later I take my car to a local garage to be serviced. Later in the afternoon while walking back to collect my car I take a short cut through a car park from Kensington Street to The Princes Highway. The level of the car park is higher than the footpath on The Princes Highway and the ground is uneven and covered with stones. I gingerly put my walking stick on the stones and step down. My walking stick slips and I fall flat on my bottom. There is nothing that I can grab to pull myself up. I struggle to get up, acutely aware of the triple lane of cars stopped at the traffic lights. The lights turn green, the cars drive off and eventually I'm back on my feet feeling very shaken. I cross the road, collect my car and drive home.

I am becoming quite unsteady on my feet and walking is painfully slow. I'm still walking to the supermarket though. I use my walking stick and I take my shopping cart. One day I'm at the supermarket checkout when the checkout girl notices that my carton of eggs is leaking. "Do you want to get another one?" she asks. I shake my head, knowing that it will take me too long to walk to the where the eggs are and I will hold everyone up. The man behind me in the queue says "I'll get you some more" and off he goes before I have a chance to write *don't bother.*

The very next day I'm on my way to post a letter. As I'm crossing the road at the traffic lights, with the green 'cross now' showing, three Chinese girls in their early 20s are crossing the road in the other direction. They walk past me and then one girl runs back to me, she grabs my arm saying "I'll help you". When we get to the other side of the road she asks "Are you OK now?" I was OK all along but these two incidents make me wonder what sort of image I'm presenting to others as I go about my daily activities.

Several days later I go to see my GP. I hand the receptionist a note saying that I want to see the doctor. Even though I've seen this doctor several times the receptionist thinks that I'm deaf and uses an elaborate series of hand movements to ask me for my Medicare card. Later I'm at the chemist shop to collect my medication. Instead of taking 2 x 25mg tablets I'm given 50mg tablets. "Now you only need to take one of these tablets. They are 50 mgs and the ones that you had before were 25 mgs and you were taking two" the lady says. She repeats the instruction and asks me if I understand. Of course I understand, I've been dealing with medication all my professional life!

I feel like saying to all these people "Hey - it's still me!" I'm not mad, deaf or helpless.

While I was in Auckland over Christmas I stopped eating porridge for breakfast. It's just too hard to manoeuvre the soft porridge around in my mouth so that I can swallow it. It just sits there on my tongue. Instead I'm having 2 x 250 ml boxes of Sanitarium 'Up & Go' for breakfast. I lost a bit of weight over the time that I was in Auckland and I mention this in an email to my dietician.

> I'm wondering if it's time I increased the amount of Jevity that I'm having.
>
> I've been losing weight. A year ago I was 56kg and last time (2 weeks ago) I weighed myself I was 47kg. I'm 151cms BMI 20.6 so that's still OK.

She replies:

> I think that we definitely need to review how much Jevity you are having. Although you are still within the desired weight range, a weight loss of almost 10kg in one year is too much. Ideally your feed regimen should keep your weight constant.

As she doesn't see outpatients the dietician makes me an appointment to see a different dietician. She tells me that I need to get a referral letter from my GP. This is crazy! I've been in contact by email with a dietician since my PEG tube was inserted in June last year and now I have to see a different person AND bring a referral letter. Surely I'm already established as a patient in the dietary department!

I arrive at the dietary department for my 2pm appointment and wait for about 20 minutes. This is the fourth dietician I've had since my PEG insertion. Although she has the nutritional plan that I was given at the time of the PEG insertion she has no idea of what has happened in the interim. I give her a typed summary of my weight, the PEG feeds that I'm having and the food I'm currently able to eat. I hop on the scales and with clothes and shoes on I'm 50 kg which is an increase of 3 kg since I weighed myself in Auckland, although really I think most of the difference is due to different scales and my clothing. Next she measures my height and with shoes on I'm 152 cm. I've gained an extra cm in height! I know that I'm 151cm.

I learn that Jevity Hi-cal has 1.5 kcal/ml and that other preparations have less kcal/ml meaning that you need to take more fluid to have the same intake of kcal. I also learn that I need 6,000-8,000 kilojoules (kj) a day to maintain my weight. I think that most of the weight that I've been losing is due to muscle wasting. From my reading I know that weight loss is a predictor of mortality but I don't really want to put any weight on. I'm going back to the dietary department to be weighed in two weeks time and I think that I'll just need to titrate my PEG feeds to keep my weight stable.

Before I move back to Auckland I have a series of final medical appointments. Firstly I see the rehab doctor. "You were moving back to Auckland in January" he says. "What happened? Did you miss the plane?" I mention to him that walking is painfully slow. "How many times have you fallen over in the past two months" he asks. 5 times. I reply. "Is your right foot catching on the ground?" Yes. "I think you need to get an AFO for your right foot." He asks me to arrange this. However, I don't think that my right foot is bad enough yet and a second AFO will only hinder my mobility. I just need to use my walking stick all the time and be more careful.

Two weeks later I go to see the respiratory doctor. The nurse weighs me and takes my vital signs. Although I've been sitting in the waiting room for 20 minutes my heart rate is up a bit at 116 beats per minutes. I think this is a reflection of the effort that it has taken me to just walk from the waiting room to the consulting room. My O2 sats are 95% which is a bit low. My blood pressure is OK though. After another wait I am seen by the registrar. I hand him my typewritten summary. He reads my summary and then listens to my chest with his stethoscope through my clothes. I wonder how well he can hear through my clothing. Then the respiratory specialist pops in to say hello and says that they will send me copies of relevant documentation about my condition to give to my new doctors in Auckland.

There are strange discoloured spots on the inside of my PEG tube that look like mould. Margie arranges for me to have the tube changed before I leave Australia. In the morning I walk over the road to the hospital to have the tube changed. The PEG nurse tells me that it isn't mould but just colonisation of the bugs in the stomach and quite normal, but it looks awful. The PEG tube is 'traction removable' which means that it can be pulled out. The pulling out requires a big pull to get the plastic bolster out through the PEG tract and it's OUCH and OUCH again!!! Inserting the new one isn't so bad because the plastic bolster is stretched out by a metal rod and it slips in through the hole in the abdominal wall.

Since I arrived back in Sydney in January I have noticed that I am having even more trouble going about my daily activities. Walking back from the shops with my groceries in my little shopping cart I often need to stop and rest. I stopped going to the gym in August but I don't think that is the reason for my deterioration. I suspect it was happening anyway. In May 2006 I had renewed my gym membership for three months with an option to extend to one year. In August, knowing that I would not be able to keep going to the gym for a whole year I didn't extend my membership. I really enjoyed the Sunday yoga/stretch/pilates class but there was no membership option where I could just attend that weekly class. As it happens my physical state has declined so much since August now there is no way that I could even manage to do the Sunday class.

I've also stopped doing my hand exercises. I didn't stop doing them intentionally. In December I was just so busy that I either didn't have time to do the hand exercises or just plain forgot to do them. While I was in Auckland my routine was too disrupted to remember to do the exercises and to be quite honest the hand exercises are boring! Back in Sydney I've been trying to remember to do them in the evening while I'm watching television but more often than not I forget.

One evening towards the end of February the Kogarah Council hosts the annual Chinese New Year concert in the Town Square opposite my apartment building. During the afternoon the sky gets darker and darker and at about 5pm it starts to rain. *Oh no!* I think. Here we are in Sydney desperately needing rain because of the drought but not tonight! About 30 minutes before the concert is due to start the rain stops. I am still eating my dinner when I hear a series of what sounds like really loud gunshots. Then I realise they are Chinese firecrackers. Next there is the sound of beating drums and I go outside and cross over to the square in time to catch the end of the Dragon dance.

Next there is a series of bi-lingual official speeches lasting about 30 minutes which is way too long! Anyway nobody can hear what is being said because all the kids are running around making a noise. The concert is a mixed bag of Chinese singing and dancing with long pauses between items as the next group gets organised.

I compare this with the Greek concert in the square in January. The Greeks were more organised.

A new restaurant/cafe/bar has just opened in the square. They have taken since before Christmas to install everything and it opens just in time for the Chinese concert. The whole inside area of the shop is taken up with the cooking and serving area. All the seating is outside on the cobblestone paving and wooden deck area. It will be lovely in the warm weather but it won't be much good in torrential rain. Maybe they are banking on continued drought. It's a pity that I can't enjoy the food and wine that the restaurant offers. All the same I'm going to miss being in the middle of all of this.

I have loved every minute of my time in Sydney, and have relished the opportunity to travel to the various hospitals in Australia and New Zealand. Looking back now, though, my travel schedule looks exhausting and I wonder how I ever managed it, though, of course I was much fitter then. In my current physical state everything is so painfully slow. Walking, dressing, eating take so long to do that the last thing that I want to do is to have to get an early morning flight for a day trip to Melbourne or Brisbane. Over the past couple of months other CRAs in the company have made trips to Amsterdam, Taiwan, Malaysia, Thailand and Korea. If I didn't have this bloody awful disease I would have been doing some of those trips.

16

A one way ticket to Auckland - March 2007

It's two weeks until I move back to Auckland. A couple of weeks ago I wrote to the real estate office giving one month's notice of vacating the apartment. Now I'm cleaning out all my drawers and cupboards and throwing lots of things away. It's amazing how much unnecessary junk I've unintentionally accumulated. In an email from a friend she asks me how I'm getting on with my moving preparations. She mentions that she has:

> ......been sorting through papers and have nearly filled a wheelie bin (one of those that you can lock and then they shred the stuff and recycle it) so that feels good.

And I reply:

> I know the feeling about going through papers! I have been going through personal and work papers and shredding them - many black plastic rubbish bags full. The shredder gets too hot and it stops. Emptying the shredder means that shredded paper ends up all over the floor as well as in the rubbish bag! So endless vacuuming! and so on ....

Every day I'm making several trips to the garbage room with big plastic rubbish bags full of shredded paper and other things. I struggle to lift the rubbish bags and take them down in the elevator and then down a flight of four tiled steps to the garbage room. I'm acutely aware of the consequences of a fall down these steps.

I'm sorting through my shoes. I have several pairs that have hardly ever been worn and they are in such good condition that I'll give them to a charity clothing shop. Although it breaks my heart, I'm throwing other shoes away. I won't ever be able to wear them again so there is no point in taking them back to Auckland. I have very small feet and I have always had trouble getting fashion shoes small enough so I have tended to hang on to my shoes longer than most people would. Now that my left foot is swollen I have only one pair of shoes that I can wear.

I'm also getting rid of blouses that need ironing. I've always found ironing to be relaxing but now I struggle to put the ironing board up and I struggle to manoeuvre the iron over my clothes. It's just so frustrating.

The real estate agent visits to take photos of the apartment to advertise it for rent on his website. "This place is as big as a two bedroom apartment" he says "and it's still like new. How long have you been here?" I hold up three fingers and then, changing my mind, hold up four. I have been here for 3 years 9 months.

It's been great! I write. "I'll miss you" he says. I'm sure he will miss me. I've been an ideal tenant, paying my rent through Rental Rewards who charge it to my Visa card.

I need to give a copy of the photo page of my passport, signed by a JP, to the removals company so I go to see the JP at the local tax consultant's office that I use here in Kogarah. It's up a very steep flight of stairs. I struggle, heaving myself up the stairs one at a time but eventually I make it to the top and get the signature that I need. Several days later I go back there again, struggling up the stairs once more, to get my final tax return done. All my payments for Jevity and medications can be claimed so this time I'm getting a refund.

I need to return the rental VPAP machine to the respiratory device company and buy my own machine. I arrange to do this and on the appointed day I struggle to disconnect the VPAP machine from the power, wind up the power cord and pack the machine, air hose and mask in the carry bag. The bag is heavy and I struggle to carry it down to my car. Arriving at the respiratory device company I am ushered into the sales rep's office. "Your machine hasn't been delivered yet" he says. *Why didn't he email me and tell me this?* I wonder. "I will get someone to drop the machine off at your place on Friday" he says. As I drive home I'm thinking *What a waste of time and effort! They just don't realise how hard it is for me to do even simple things like packing up and carrying the machine.*

At home, I unpack the rental machine and set it up again. Friday comes and there is no sign of the sales rep or the new machine. So I send an email.

> Sorry he couldn't make it. Would you like to come and collect it on Monday at 10am? is the response.

Monday comes and now I have Dylan with me. Dylan packs up the VPAP machine for me and we drive over to the company's office again. On arrival I report to the receptionist. "He hasn't come in today - his son is sick" she says. She asks if I would like to wait for another rep to drive over from Westmead which is 1½ hours drive away or would I like to come back tomorrow? I have things to do tomorrow so we wait. After about an hour or so a lady comes in and is given the same message, "the rep isn't here." This lady makes a fuss and the manager comes out and deals with her. I write a note to the receptionist *Why is she seen first? I've been waiting longer?* I'm angry about being ignored. Just then the rep from Westmead arrives and attends to me. It's hopeless though. I'm buying a $7,000 machine from them and I'm treated as if I don't matter! I haven't even received an emailed apology from the original rep!

I need to sell all of my furniture. I take photos of the things I want to sell and Dylan and I put notices up in all the apartment buildings in the street. Before long people phone us and come to view the items for sale. We take deposits and arrange for the people to return on Thursday to pay the balance and collect their purchases. By Thursday we have sold all the small and medium sized items and my bed.

On Thursday morning the movers arrive and move through the place like a tornado, packing things. Before I realise it, they have packed up quite a few of the things that I want to put in my luggage. It's too late now though, the boxes are sealed. When the movers have packed everything we are left with the lounge suite, dining table, outside table and chairs, fridge and washing machine. One of the movers asks Dylan if we want to sell them. I have been offered $300 for the lot by one of the second hand shops in Rockdale but it's worth much more than that. Dylan says the movers, who are three Maori guys from Northland, are all "good guys" and he would rather I sold it to him than to the shop in Rockdale who will only re-sell it for double the price. So by the end of the day everything is packed or sold, except for the car.

On February 15 I wrote a letter to the car finance company advising them that as I am leaving the country I will be selling my car and asking how I can pay the balance owing on the loan. On March 1st, having received no reply to my letter, I send an email:

> I wish to advise you that I will be leaving Australia permanently on March 10.
> I need to pay the balance owing on my car before selling it.
> Please send me a statement of payments made to date and the balance owing.
> Please advise me how I can pay the balance.
> I am contacting you by email rather than by phone as I have lost my voice permanently due to a medical condition.
> Please respond by email.

And the following day, having received no response, I send another email:

> Please advise me when I can expect a response to my request below. I am selling my car.

I received 'read receipts' for both emails, so I know that they were received and read but I had no response to the letter or the emails. By the time Dylan arrives I'm getting desperate. On Monday Dylan phones the car finance company, explaining that his Mum has lost her voice and he is calling on her behalf. After a prolonged call, being kept on 'hold' for a lot of the time and being transferred from one person to another he is advised "We will post a letter to your Mother. It won't be posted until tomorrow." On Wednesday we anxiously check the mail box but no letter arrives.

On Thursday Dylan phones the finance company again. He explains again that I need to pay off the loan as I am leaving the country on Saturday. He emphasizes that this requires URGENT attention. They agree to fax something to me if I agree to pay $16 for the fax!!

It's Friday and still no fax has arrived. I need to sell my car today. Dylan phones the finance company again. The person he speaks to is unhelpful and we are no further ahead. In desperation, I ask Dylan to phone my boss and ask him if he could phone the finance company. My boss duly phones the company and gets the same protracted treatment of being placed on hold and transferred from one person to another. Eventually, by threatening to contact the person's supervisor, my boss is given an undertaking that a fax will be sent within the hour. Sure enough I receive a fax within about 10 minutes.

The fax contains all the information that I need: the amount owing on the car and the BPAY code needed to pay it at the Post Office. A little later on Friday the letter arrives in the mail. It has the amount owing on the loan but not the BPAY code. Why was this so hard? Why didn't the company respond to my initial letter sent on 15 February? Why didn't they respond to my emails sent on 1 and 2 March? When I'm back in Auckland I'm going to submit an official complaint to the managing director of the company.

Dylan phones the car sales company he had spoken to earlier in the week. Within an hour two guys come and check out the car. They are happy with it and pay me cash on the spot. Phew! Everything is sold, packed, cleaned, cancelled, closed and I'm ready to go. We take a taxi to the Novotel at Brighton-le-Sands for our final night in Sydney.

On Saturday morning I take a taxi to the local chemist shop in Kogarah to collect all the rest of my medication. Then I stop at the real estate office and drop off the keys to the apartment.

Back at the hotel I re-pack my suitcases and we are on our way to the airport.

My baggage weighs 60 kgs and even with Dylan's baggage allowance it is way over weight. But the lady at the Qantas check in recognises the I've lost my voice written on the top of my ticket and she says that she won't charge me excess baggage. "I remember your Mum, she's a sweetie" she says to Dylan. We move on through passport control and security, Dylan buys some duty free things, I buy some duty free perfume for Emma's birthday and then we wait in the Qantas Club until it's time to board our flight to Auckland.

Dylan has been such a great help over the past week, I really couldn't have managed without him. I have been so busy focusing on the things that I have had to do that I haven't had time to feel sad about moving. But I know that I'm really going to miss living in Sydney and the lifestyle that I've had. I've had wonderful support from family and friends, most of whom have managed to visit me while I've been in Sydney and see for themselves how good everything has been. This email from a friend says it all:

> Hope your move goes as well as can be hoped – it will indeed be a major jolt after what has been a very successful stint in Sydney both professionally and personally.